Globalization and Integration of Internationally Educated Nurses: A Comprehensive Analysis

Rola El Moubadder • Ruth Wojtiuk
Ruth Lee
Editors

Globalization and Integration of Internationally Educated Nurses: A Comprehensive Analysis

Springer

Editors
Rola El Moubadder
CARE Centre for Internationally
Educated Nurses
Toronto, ON, Canada

Ruth Wojtiuk
CARE Centre for Internationally
Educated Nurses
Toronto, ON, Canada

Ruth Lee
CARE Centre for Internationally
Educated Nurses
Toronto, ON, Canada

ISBN 978-3-032-01105-3 ISBN 978-3-032-01106-0 (eBook)
https://doi.org/10.1007/978-3-032-01106-0

This Springer imprint is published by the registered company Springer Nature Switzerland AG
The registered company address is: Gewerbestrasse 11, 6330 Cham, Switzerland

Foreword

This book is important and well-conceived.

Why Is It Important?

It draws attention to international migration, which is at its highest levels in human history. The United Nations estimates that international migration comprised 3.5% (281 million) of the global population in 2020, compared to 2.8% in 2000 and 2.3% in 1980. The UN identifies this phenomenon as a global issue that is driven by both individual choice and individual/family/group necessity (https://www.un.org/en/global-issues/migration).

In this context of international migration, the unique importance of this book derives from its detailed documentation of how programs are responding to the complex issues and the opportunities for internationally qualified nurses in five migrant-receiving nations.

What Makes the Structure of This Book Well-Conceived?

It showcases the experience and learning in these five countries, and analyzes the variety of ways in which they receive and induct internationally qualified nurses into professional practice.

These are reflective ground-level perspectives. Through the voices of front-line staff and program managers, this book provides first-person description, testimonial, and analysis of the strategies and programs being employed to receive and support internationally educated nurses in their new country of residence.

This granular multi-country comparative examination fosters a deep understanding of the issues faced by migrating nurses and shares perspectives on the efficacy, and the evolution, of solutions. The solutions differ from country to country, but it is clear that they have a common goal: To enable these newcomers to quickly and efficiently maximize their professional contribution within our healthcare system.

These authors are brilliant, have well-grounded insights, and will introduce you to new conceptual and practical frameworks and strategies that work.

You are in good hands.

Phil Schalm has focused on supporting immigrant professionals in Canada during the past several decades, and has developed and delivered programs in healthcare and other sectors that bridge them to professional licensure and successful careers in Canada. Currently, he is chair of the board of directors for The CARE Centre For Internationally Educated Nurses.

Chair Board of Directors, Toronto, Ontario, Canada Phil Schalm

Foreword

Nursing is a global profession, with an estimated total workforce of almost 30 million nurses worldwide (World Health Organization 2025). Nurses offer significant expertise wherever they are employed and regardless of the level of autonomy they exercise within their roles, which also makes nurses highly sought worldwide. Nursing is indeed a hyper-mobile profession, with global distribution patterns showing continued international mobility and migration (World Health Organization 2025). These international trends highlight the timeliness of this book: *Globalization and Integration of Internationally Educated Nurses: A Comprehensive Analysis*.

In Canada, there is widespread support for Internationally Educated Nurses (IENs). The *Nursing Retention Toolkit* (Health Canada 2024) highlights strategies for effective integration of IENs into our Canadian health care systems. Yet, there is always more to be done to better integrate IENs and support their transition to the Canadian healthcare context. Readers of this book can benefit from learning about the international case studies and success stories presented herein.

IENs offer valuable contributions to the Canadian health workforce and Canada is better for its diverse nursing workforce, which mirrors the diversity of the Canadian population. I applaud El Moubadder, Wojtiuk, and Lee for their significant contributions to the work of integrating and transitioning IENs within Canada and thank them for compiling their expertise on this topic in this book. I encourage readers to consider nurse migration as a phenomenon that is not soon to disappear and to heed the recommendations on IEN transition supports and integration wherever possible. The topic of IENs in global nursing workforce policy and planning is an important contemporary issue which makes this book's focus extremely prescient.

References

Health Canada. Nursing Retention Toolkit: Improving the working lives of nurses in Canada. 2024. Available at: Canada.ca/NursingToolkit.
World Health Organization. State of the world's nursing 2025: investing in education, jobs, leadership and service delivery. Geneva. 2025.

Leigh Chapman
Canada's Chief Nurse Office (CNO), Health Canada
Ottawa, ON, Canada

Introduction

Global migration in the contemporary world represents around 258 million international migrants. Today people are moving more than ever before. That figure has grown rapidly since the turn of the millennium when there were 173 million. Together with the increasing volume, we are seeing changing demographics, advancing technology, evolving needs of labor markets, and continued challenges posed by wars, shortages, human rights violations, and climate change. We sometimes think of certain countries as sources of migrants and others as recipients. But most nations today experience migration from all three perspectives—as countries of origin, transit, and destination [1].

Humanity has always been on the move. Throughout history, we have migrated in search of new opportunities, as well as to escape persecution, conflict, and poverty. Movements of people happen all around the world. Although migration is a global phenomenon, there is still limited global understanding of how to manage it [1]. Countries at all levels of socioeconomic development face, to varying degrees, difficulties in the employment, deployment, retention, and performance of their immigrant nursing workforce [2].

Amid persistent health workforce shortages and increasing global demand for skilled professionals, migration has become a cornerstone strategy for addressing gaps in care and building resilient healthcare systems. The migration of nurses and other healthcare professionals has continued to shape healthcare workforces worldwide in 2024 as governments work to prop up struggling healthcare systems amid persistent staffing shortages [3].

Drawing on the evidence based best practices of magnet countries Canada, the USA, Finland, Australia, and the United Kingdom, this volume is designed for academics, policymakers, healthcare leaders, employers, and stakeholders invested in workforce planning,

Throughout the chapters, countries will consistently analyze their experiences, reflecting on the impact of the global nursing shortage as it relates to the national healthcare context. Remediation efforts focusing on immigration policies, licensure pathways, and employment supports will be examined along with recommendations to meet the present and future challenges surrounding recruitment approaches, integration strategies, and retention initiatives. All aimed at providing actionable insights to inform policy, improve workforce strategies, promote sustainable healthcare solutions, and equip stakeholders with a menu of tools to help navigate the complexities of nurse migration and advance collaborative, ethical solutions for workforce sustainability.

References

1. World Economic forum Jan 10, 2020. "Jobs and the future of work" Global migration, by the numbers: who migrates, where they go and why.
2. WHO Health workforce international platform on health worker mobility.
3. Nurse Migration report February 11 2024 A report by CGFNS International, Inc.

Contents

Streamlining Integration and Licensure: Strategies to Capture the Contribution of International Nurses to the Canadian Healthcare System

Rola El Moubadder, Ruth Lee, and Ruth Wojtiuk

Global Nursing Shortage and Its Impact on Canadian Health Human Resources

In 2009, the Canadian Nurses Association projected a nursing shortage of 60,000 registered nurses (RNs) by 2022. This prediction had been surpassed, as the shortage is more severe because of the high demand for nurses during the COVID-19 pandemic and is expected to worsen over the period of 2022–2031 at the national level [17, 18]. The shortage is even more acute in historically recruitment challenged remote and rural Canada [37]. One-third of nurses (30.3%) reported working overtime, nearly double the proportion of 15.7% reported in 1997. Nurses are exhausted from overwork and very stressful practice environments, which resulted in a high degree of absenteeism due to illness or disability [9]; many are contemplating leaving the profession [7]. The recent increase in Canadian-educated nurses has been marginal and is insufficient to fill all the nursing vacancies projected across Canada [4]. Despite these human resource challenges, only 69% of internationally educated nurses (IENs) were employed in health occupations compared to 87% of Canadian-educated nurses [17]. The COVID-19 pandemic has certainly accentuated the nursing shortage and brought it to the forefront of national attention, but the nursing shortage has been a long-standing issue in the past two decades. In this section, contributing factors that led to the current critical state of the Canadian nursing shortage, government, and nursing leaders' strategies in ameliorating the shortage, as well as potential solutions, including capitalizing on the contribution of IENs, are discussed.

R. El Moubadder (✉) · R. Lee · R. Wojtiuk
CARE Centre for Internationally Educated Nurses, Toronto, ON, Canada
e-mail: rmoubadder@care4nurses.org; rlee@care4nurses.org; rwojtiuk@care4nurses.org;
https://www.care4nurses.org; https://www.care4nurses.org; https://www.care4nurses.org

R. El Moubadder et al. (eds.), *Globalization and Integration of Internationally Educated Nurses: A Comprehensive Analysis*,
https://doi.org/10.1007/978-3-032-01106-0_1

Contributing Factors to the Canadian Nursing Shortage

Historically, the nursing shortage in Canada has been a complex issue with multiple interconnected factors that include demographic changes in our population, working conditions and compensation, government policies, barriers in the regulatory process for IENs, and biases in employer hiring practices.

Demographic Changes with Increasing Diversity

Canada is a multicultural and multilingual country with over one hundred ethnocultural groups represented; nearly 25% of Canadians are foreign-born [54]. In 2010, Statistics Canada predicted that immigrants would constitute 28% of Canada's population by 2031 [55]. Since the beginning of the 1990s, immigration has been the key driver of population growth in Canada; in the first quarter of 2024, 99.3% (240, 955) of our population growth was from new immigrants [52]. To rebuild Canada's post-pandemic economy and sustain our workforce because of an aging population and low birth rate, the government has increased the level of annual immigration target to an unprecedented level of 485,000 in 2024, 500,000 in 2025, and stabilized it at 500,000 in 2026 [40]. Unlike the early European settlers of the Nation, many of our newcomers are from India, the Philippines, and other Asian and some African countries. Most of these newcomers do not have English or French (official languages of Canada) as their first language, and neither do they share the Western cultural values and health practices of the larger Canadian population. The majority are professionals with specialized skills and a high level of education; they migrate to Canada through the multiple immigration pathways created by the government to accelerate their application process so that they can meet the human resource needs of post-pandemic Canada. Many are immigrating with their immediate and extended families. Despite the recent increase in the number of immigrants, the high rate of retention among the 4- to 7-year post-arrival cohort presents a significant issue. Also of concern is that many of those leaving the country are younger newcomers [21, 34]. This pattern begs the question of the effectiveness of our retention strategies. With the increasing population comes the higher demand for health services, which adds to the shortage of nurses. While new immigrants increase the linguistic and ethnocultural diversities of the Canadian population, to date, the Canadian nursing workforce remains largely homogenous and does not represent the increasingly diverse Canadian population [39]; we need healthcare workers who are prepared to provide culturally appropriate care in languages that reflect the patient populations they serve. Healthcare organizations need nurse innovators with international experience, new insights, and linguistic and cultural expertise to provide culturally sensitive patient-centered care.

Aging Population

The share of people aged 65 and older within the total population would increase from 18.9% in 2023, and those aged 85 and older are projected to triple by 2073. Older people require more health care, thus creating a greater demand for nursing services; however, the number of nurses who provide direct care decreased from 59 per 1,000 older adults in 2013 to 52 per 1,000 in 2022 [52]. In the long-term care sector, there was a 5.1% decline in the nursing supply from 2021 to 2022 [17]. As the Canadian population is aging, so is our nursing workforce. At a time when our aging population and high chronic illness prevalence create a high demand for nursing care, the number of nurses retiring is higher than the number of new graduates [2]. This situation intensifies the nursing shortage.

IENs' Challenges in Licensing and Workplace Integration Worsen Nursing Shortage

Approximately 10% of Canada's regulated nurses have been educated abroad, an increase of 2% since 2013; in 2022, 12% of newly licensed nurses were IENs [17]. Despite being perceived as an untapped resource in easing the shortage, they encounter multiple challenges in transitioning and integrating into the Canadian workforce. These challenges include verifying the equivalency of credentials; obtaining registration, securing, and retaining employment; and overcoming cultural and communication barriers [20, 35, 38, 47].

Despite overcoming all the barriers and obtaining their Canadian license, IENs face challenges in obtaining commensurate employment, as employers are skeptical in hiring IENs [4]. IENs are also severely underemployed, as 69% of nurse aides, orderlies, and patient service associates are IENs with a nursing degree [57]. Most IENs are RNs in their home countries, but through evaluation of their credentials by regulatory bodies, they are deemed equivalent to a registered practical nurse (RPN). Although they are contributing, they are limited in using all their expertise, thus hindering both their career mobility and advancement [51].

A scoping review conducted by the Canadian Nurses Association revealed evidence of the racism and discrimination experienced by nurses from ethnic minority backgrounds across all domains of practice in Canada [18]. Compared with their Anglo-Saxon counterparts, job applicants who have "foreign-sounding" last names are not as likely to be called for an interview [3]. Effective integration requires nurse managers and nurses to be aware of these issues and commit to promoting cultural diversity in the workplace [28, 32].

Strategies in Meliorating the Shortage

To ease the current shortage and retain and sustain the nursing workforce, nursing leaders are calling for urgent changes in our healthcare system and to address organizational barriers, particularly in improving the working environment and allowing nurses to practice to their full scope of practice [7]. A healthier work environment for nurses would ultimately improve care for patients. The role of the National Chief Nursing Officer was reinstated in August 2022 after being vacant for almost a decade. A nursing retention plan led by the Chief Nursing Officer is part of the government's investment of more than $200 billion over 10 years to improve health care for Canadians. The plan, accompanied by a toolkit with practical strategies and tools to improve the retention of nurses, has been developed for nurse employers, healthcare organizations, and health system administrators [26]. The federal government also provides funding to the Canadian Association of Schools of Nursing, which represents baccalaureate and graduate nursing programs across Canada, to support the integration and retention of IENs in the workforce [11]. Policies and initiatives supporting IEN recruitment, transition, and integration are being strengthened and offered by federal and provincial governments [5, 58].

Government Policies in Recruitment and Retention

Multiple policies, some built on existing new graduate transition and retention initiatives, have been enacted to address the national staffing crisis in all healthcare service sectors. Despite Canada's long-standing policy commitment to the International Council of Nurses' [30] position that "wealthy countries" need to be self-sufficient in their nursing workforce and not to recruit from other countries, international recruitment reached an all-time high in 2021, particularly for less populated areas where healthcare employers were confronted with a serious shortage. It is expected that international recruitment will continue to increase as the federal and provincial governments enact policies that enable or facilitate ethical international recruitment [44] to meet patient care needs.

Unprecedented rapid policy changes and mandates from the government to regulatory bodies resulted in many barriers confronting IENs being removed, and the licensing processes expedited [17]. Notably, the language test requirement was removed for native English speakers and substantially reduced for English as a second-language speaker. Language competence can be met by evidence of working in an English-speaking workplace with verification by management/coworkers or through a formal language test.

Program to Expedite Immigration Applicants with Healthcare Background

The federal government invites individuals with healthcare expertise to immigrate to Canada through Express Entry with "healthcare occupations" at the top of the categories [24] and sets higher targets for Provincial Nominee Programs to allow provinces to have immigration streams for healthcare workers, including nurses, to make their immigration process streamlined and faster [25].

Increase in Educational Opportunities and Financial Support

Some provinces have increased the number of seats in their education and bridge training programs to help IENs meet the educational gaps identified by regulators. Reimbursement of expenses (tuition for training and courses, assessment and exams, licensing, and registration costs) associated with the licensure process is provided to IENs who have successfully registered. Bridging and upskilling programs are available to IENs across the country (such as the BEGIN initiative in Ontario and Alberta's Bursary for the IEN program), but IENs must first pay for expenses and then be reimbursed, which poses financial challenges for the IENs. Financial incentives are also offered to IENs to work in rural and remote areas in several provinces and territories.

Individualized Navigation Services

Nurse Navigator models have been implemented in some provinces to help IENs navigate the assessment and licensure processes. The CARE Centre for Internationally Educated Nurses' (Pre-arrival Supports and Service (PASS) program, funded by the federal government, provides IENs in their countries of residence who are planning immigration to Canada with one-on-one case management support, educational webinars, and mentorship in collaboration with the Canadian Nurses Association. The CARE Centre's Supports, Training, and Access to Regulated-employment Services program (STARS), funded by the Ontario government, supports IENs with one-on-one case management; language and communication training; examination preparation; professional development; a mentorship program in partnership with employers and professional associations; and networking to prepare IENs to relaunch their nursing careers in Canada [19].

Regulatory and Licensing Requirement Changes

Some provinces have signed Memorandum of Understandings (MOUs) with the Philippines and India to streamline and expedite the registration process for nurses from these countries. The Temporary Class licensure for nurses introduced in

Ontario allows nurses to practice with some limitations in their scope of practice; meeting the language requirements is no longer limited to specific language tests but can include feedback from supervisors and coworkers in some provinces.

Registration Examination Eligibility Requirements

Some provinces deem IENs to meet their competency requirements if they have passed the National Council Licenser Examination (NCLEX) in another jurisdiction, registered in other Canadian provinces, or are educated in countries that are deemed equivalent to Canada. Nova Scotia's expedited registration and licensure process resulted in an increase of 9.25% for IENs from designated countries within 6 months of its launch on May 1, 2023 [42]. British Columbia also introduced an IEN Pilot Pathway on January 30, 2023, which shortened the total time of the registration assessment phase from 2 to 5 years to 2 to 10 months [8].

Additional Options to Meet Current Practice Requirement

Practice experience within a 3-year time frame is one of the requirements for registration for nursing. IENs who lapsed this time frame are required to refresh their current practice to obtain their registration, and many would return to their home country to practice for a mandated period to meet this requirement. Based on a successful pilot project conducted by the CARE Centre and its employer partners, the Province of Ontario and the College of Nurses of Ontario launched the Supervised Practice Experience Program (SPEP) as an additional option to refresh their current practice without leaving the province. Employers' evaluation of the SPEP has been a positive component of their recruitment and retention strategies for IENs and indicates that they contribute significantly to equity, diversity, and inclusivity in the workplace [31].

Migration of IENs

A shrinking supply of health human resources and rising demand for health services have put health systems around the world at a crucial crossroads. Even though COVID-19 worsened nurse shortages, it was clear decades ago that Canada's health human resources needed to be strengthened and maintained, as evidenced by multiple studies that warned of severe shortages. Building the capacity of the health system has become critical since the pandemic. The creative nurse employment initiatives in Canada are examined in this section and throughout the book. Federal, provincial, and territorial policies/strategies are enacted with an emphasis on IENs in light of the growing demand for and global competition for their services and expertise. However, more measures are recommended in recognition of the ongoing difficulty of health human resource planning. Among these is the creation of complementary policies to enhance IEN mobilization, sustainable recruitment, and workforce integration.

Ben-Ahmed HE et al. in their article referred to government-led initiatives and nongovernmental and nursing-led initiatives that are key to building the strategy to pan-Canadian nursing workforce recruitment and retention referring to reports from 1999 to 2022. From the reports discussed in the article, the federal government has illustrated instrumental initiative such as the "Nursing strategy for Canada" in 2000 under federal initiatives and "CFNU's report on healthy workplaces" in 2001 under nongovernmental initiatives. Additionally, in 2024, there were two published work, "Scoping Review by the Canadian Nurse Association" and "Health Canada under the CNO initiative developed Nursing Retention Toolkit," that aligned with the ongoing efforts of both the federal governmental initiatives and the nongovernmental nursing-led initiatives. These instrumental contributions reflect the sustained efforts to strengthen nursing capacity, address workforce challenges, and integrate internationally educated nurses (IENs) into the healthcare system. On the federal side, significant policy developments from the Nursing Strategy for Canada (2000) and Pan-Canadian Health Human Resources Strategy (2004/2007) to the more recent 2022 federal CNO appointment and funding for nursing education that highlight a long-term commitment to workforce planning, regulation, and support for IEN integration. These actions aim to improve licensure pathways, ensure safer working conditions, and enhance data collection on nurses' work environments and health.

Collectively, these initiatives reflect a comprehensive approach to building workforce capacity by aligning policy, research, and practical interventions. They also increasingly recognize the importance of including IENs in workforce planning, addressing barriers to their integration, and leveraging their contributions to meet Canada's healthcare needs in the face of global nursing shortages [6].

Recruitment

The Government of Canada has a strict policy in place, emphasizing the ethical international recruitment of health professionals, specifically nurses. In adherence to international standards, the Canadian approach aligns with the World Health Organization (WHO)'s Global Code of Practice on the International Recruitment of Health Personnel, which aims to avoid "brain drain" and minimize the adverse impact of active recruitment from nations with critical health workforce shortages. While protecting both the source country's nursing workforce and the individual rights of recruits, Canada stresses the key principles of voluntary international recruitment of nurses, transparency, and fair recruitment practices. Recruitment agencies, employers, and health authorities are expected to operate within fair and transparent hiring practices, providing IENs with accurate and clear information about job roles, wages, and working conditions and protecting them from exploitation [26, 27].

Both federal and provincial governments have launched several programs aiming to attract and recruit IENs. These initiatives aim to address the nursing shortage crisis, as IENs being recognized to bring talents and skills in specialized areas. Despite the government's commitment to streamlining the immigration and licensing pathways, IENs still face challenges in navigating the most suitable avenues that allow them to obtain permanent residency, secure employment in nursing, and smooth integration. Like many developed countries, Canada tends to rely heavily on international nurse mobility and migration to compensate for a short supply of domestic nursing graduates (The WHO Global Strategic Directions for Nursing and Midwifery, 2021–2025). Canadian governments at the federal, provincial, and territorial levels are looking at creating recruitment strategies and nursing employment programs to mitigate the nursing shortage, with an emphasis on IENs in light of the growing demand for and competition for their services and skills. However, more initiatives are recommended in recognition of the ongoing difficulty of health human resource planning, such as policy frameworks that support proactive long-term strategies to address the cyclical shortage of nurses and complementary policy development to improve the retention of IENs.

To assist IENs in overcoming barriers to having their credentials recognized and lowering the time and cost, the Foreign Credential Recognition Program (FCRP), through provincial and territorial government funds, helps IENs pay for the expenses of licensing, exams, and language training. By reducing the time and cost barriers, this initiative expedites the integration of IENs into the workforce. The FCRP is overseen by Employment and Social Development Canada (ESDC) (Government of Canada, [24, 25]). For example, Canada recently launched a new pathway under the *Temporary Resident to Permanent Resident Pathway* for healthcare workers, allowing those on temporary visas to transition to permanent residency. Some provinces took advantage of such initiatives, such as Manitoba, leveraging the Temporary Foreign Worker Program (TFWP) in health care to recruit nurses on a temporary basis. Although this program is temporary, it provides an immediate solution to fill critical gaps in healthcare services. Many nurses who come to Canada under the TFWP later transition to permanent residency through other immigration pathways. Another initiative is Quebec's Permanent Immigration Pilot Program, which specifically targets foreign-trained nurses, offering an expedited route to residency for healthcare professionals [29]. Most of the recruitment initiatives are provincially led with the support of the federal government, but owing to variations in nursing demand and the regulatory process among provinces, these initiatives are inconsistent and sometimes are short-term fix to the nursing shortages rather than offering sustainable and consistent national solutions. British Columbia invested in supporting IENs through British Columbia's Newcomer Program for Healthcare Workers. This program helps IENs in their credential recognition process and connects them with job opportunities in the province [8].

However, supporting IEN recruitment has alleviated some of the pressures faced by hospitals and clinics, particularly in urban areas. Hospitals in large cities have seen more staffing flexibility and a better distribution of nurses, leading to improved patient care and reduced wait times in some areas. Rural communities continue to face nursing shortages, as recruitment efforts often do not address the long-term support and integration needed to retain nurses in remote locations. This limits the effectiveness of initiatives in achieving equitable healthcare access across the country. When reviewing Canada's recruitment trends, the data indicate that IENs had a considerably lower likelihood of pursuing careers that aligned with their educational background in comparison to those who completed programs within Canada. For example, compared with 78% of immigrants who finished their education in Canada, only 37% of immigrants who completed a bachelor's degree or higher in a nursing program outside of Canada were employed in these occupations [17, 52, 53].

Overall, the government's initiatives to recruit IENs have achieved short-term gains by filling vacancies, increasing workforce diversity, and supporting the rapid integration of IENs into the healthcare system. However, ongoing challenges in rural retention, systemic workplace pressures, and regional disparities limit the full effectiveness of these initiatives. Long-term success will likely require continued investment in nursing retention, broader workplace reforms, and targeted incentives for service in rural and underserved areas to ensure sustainable workforce stability.

In the immigration policies section, the key government immigration programs and pathways are illustrated in detail.

Immigration Policies and Pathways

Canada offers several recent immigration pathways to immigrants that are specifically tailored to nurses and healthcare providers. Candidate immigrants are assessed differently on the basis of the immigration stream they apply through. Some immigration streams, such as Express Entry, assess candidates to determine eligibility for permanent residency based on the Comprehensive Ranking System (CSR) point-based system and the National Occupational Classification (NOC) system within Training, Education, Experience, and Responsibilities (TEER). Whatever immigration pathway a candidate has been assessed against, candidates' age, education, work experience, language proficiency, and other factors will be evaluated to determine eligibility to process their temporary or permanent residency, as well as meeting the Canada's admissibility requirements, including security, criminality, and medical checks [29]. IENs might choose to migrate to Canada through the various immigration pathways listed and described in Table 1

While the federal government provides several immigration programs, as indicated, not all pathways offer immigrants permanent residency, allowing them to gain work permits.

Most immigration pathways are not designed in a way that facilitates credentialing and licensing of the IENs, and there is a disconnect between the immigration pathways and the regulatory bodies on the provincial side as well as the healthcare system [23].

These programs collectively help skilled workers, caregivers, entrepreneurs, and family members immigrate and contribute to Canada's economy and society [29].

Table 1 A summary of the key immigration pathways available in Canada [24, 25, 29]

Immigration pathways	Categories/eligibility criteria	Work permit and permanent residency status
Express Entry: It is a fast-track system for skilled workers. It manages applications for three programs [24]	*Eligibility*: Based on a points system (Comprehensive Ranking System [CRS]) where candidates are assessed on age, education, work experience, language proficiency, and other factors. Candidates with the highest CRS scores are invited to apply for permanent residence through periodic draws from the Express Entry pool *Federal Skilled Worker Program (FSWP)*: Eligible candidates require at least 1 year of full-time work experience within the last 10 years [24] *Federal Skilled Trades Program (FSTP)*: Eligible candidates require a minimum of 2 years of full-time work experience (or an equal amount of part-time experience) in a skilled trade within the last 5 years. Some examples of skilled trades include electricians, plumbers, and carpenters *Canadian Experience Class (CEC)*: For those candidates with at least 1 year of full-time Canadian skilled work experience within the last 3 years	*Permanent residency*: Candidates with high scores receive invitations to apply for permanent residency. Express Entry is focused on permanent residency, but applicants can enter on a temporary work permit while their application is processed *Work permit*: Not directly tied to Express Entry, but applicants often need valid Canadian work experience or a job offer for additional CRS points [24]

(continued)

Table 1 (continued)

Immigration pathways	Categories/eligibility criteria	Work permit and permanent residency status
Provincial Nominee Program (PNP): Provinces and territories can nominate immigrants based on their individual skills, education, and work experience to contribute to economy and local labor market needs. Some streams target healthcare professionals like nurses such as employer job offer, employer, and job offer foreign worker [25]	*Eligibility*: Varies by province; typically requires job offers, specific skills in demand, or work experience in a specific occupation. Each province or territory has its own streams and requirements tailored to its economic needs [25]	*Permanent residency*: PNP nominates candidates for permanent residency. After nomination, applicants can apply through the federal system for permanent residency. Some PNP streams allow for temporary residency or work permits while waiting for permanent residency processing *Work permit*: In many cases, a job offer from a provincial employer is required for eligibility [25]
Family sponsorship: Canadian citizens and permanent residents can sponsor relatives, such as spouses, children, parents, and grandparents, to immigrate to Canada [29]	*Eligibility*: Requires a Canadian citizen or permanent resident to sponsor eligible family members, such as spouses, children, parents, or grandparents [29]	*Permanent residency*: Once nominated, individuals can apply to Immigration Refugee Citizenship Canada for permanent residents. Family sponsorship typically focuses on permanent residency, though temporary permits may apply while processing *Work permit*: Spouses can apply for open work permits while waiting for permanent residency [29]

(continued)

Table 1 (continued)

Immigration pathways	Categories/eligibility criteria	Work permit and permanent residency status
Start-up visa: For entrepreneurs who have the skills to build innovative business in Canada. The business could be supported by a designated Canadian organization to create jobs for Canadian [29]	*Eligibility*: Requires a qualifying business supported by a designated Canadian organization, along with language proficiency and settlement funds [29]	*Permanent residency*: Successful entrepreneurs receive permanent residency upon approval of their business plan and visa application *Work permit*: Applicants can apply for a temporary work permit to start their business in Canada while their permanent residency application is being processed. Work permits provide temporary residency status during the processing phase [29]
Caregivers: Canada offers pathways for caregivers to become permanent residents after working in Canada through specific programs, including home support and childcare provider roles. Most IENs from Philippine migrate under this stream [29]	*Eligibility*: Caregivers must have Canadian work experience in home care or childcare under a temporary work permit The two primary programs are: *Home child care provider and home support pilot* Candidates must have a job offer in Canada as a home childcare provider or have previously worked in Canada in this role. Accumulate at least 12 months of full-time work experience as a home childcare provider within the last 36 months. Each pilot has an annual cap of 2,750 principal applicants [29]	*Permanent residency*: After completing the qualifying Canadian work experience, caregivers can apply for permanent residency. Caregivers hold temporary work permits during their qualifying work period. Caregivers and their immediate families can apply for permanent residence through these pilots, provided they meet the eligibility criteria *Work permit*: Caregivers start with a temporary work permit and must work in Canada to be eligible for permanent residency [29]

(continued)

Table 1 (continued)

Immigration pathways	Categories/eligibility criteria	Work permit and permanent residency status
Agri-food pilot: This is a targeted program to address labor shortages in Canada's agriculture and food sectors, particularly in meat processing, mushroom production, and other high-demand areas. The pilot has an annual cap of 2,750 applications [29]	*Eligibility*: Requires experience in specific agri-food industries (e.g., meat processing and mushroom farming), a job offer, and basic language proficiency [29]	*Permanent residency*: Workers in the agri-food sector can apply for permanent residency after accumulating fulfilling the program's criteria. Workers often start as temporary residents under the program while their permanent residency is processed Work permit: Initially, workers may need a temporary work permit to gain the necessary experience [29]
Rural and Northern Immigration Pilot will be expanding to Rural Community Immigration Francophone Community Immigration Pilot: This program was a community-driven aimed at attracting skilled foreign workers. It is aimed at filling labor shortages in rural areas [29]	*Eligibility*: Requires a job offer in a participating rural or northern community and meeting specific criteria (education, work experience, and language skills) [29]	*Permanent residency*: Candidates become eligible for permanent residency upon fulfilling program requirements. Applicants can hold temporary residency status (via work permits) while waiting for permanent residency. At least 1 year of continuous full-time work experience (or equivalent part-time experience) in a skilled occupation within the last 3 years *Work permit*: Job offers usually require applicants to have or apply for temporary work permits [29]

(continued)

Table 1 (continued)

Immigration pathways	Categories/eligibility criteria	Work permit and permanent residency status
Atlantic Immigration Program (AIP): It is designed to attract skilled workers and international graduates to Canada's Atlantic provinces: New Brunswick, Newfoundland and Labrador, Nova Scotia, and Prince Edward Island [29]	*Eligibility*: Candidates obtain a full-time, nonseasonal job offer from a designated employer in one of the Atlantic provinces. The job offer must be for a position you are qualified to perform and intend to carry out. This stream includes certain healthcare sector jobs. the job offer does not need to be at the same skill level as your qualifying work experience [29]	*Permanent residency*: Candidates require at least 1 year of full-time (or equivalent part-time) work experience in the last 5 years in a skilled occupation The work experience must include most of the main duties listed in the National Occupational Classification (NOC) for that occupation Candidates express a genuine intention to live in the Atlantic province that endorses their application [29]

The Most Common IEN Pathways

The pathways that target IENs and are tailored to meet the needs of the nursing workforce are the Express Entry and Provincial Nominee Programs (PNP). IENs often score higher through point-based systems because of their education, work experience, and language proficiency. Moreover, these programs provide a faster route to permanent residency and are particularly useful for recruiting nurses to underserved or rural areas. The majority of IENs from the Philippines are authorized immigrants under either Express Entry or caregivers immigration streams, the majority of whom are principal candidates. Half of them were accepted under initiatives that provide a route to permanent residency for those who are in the caregiver category. Seventy-five (75) percent of immigrants who immigrated from the Philippines as nurses held the highest level of education in nursing before arriving in Canada [54]. Adding to this, all those who migrate regardless of the immigration program may have completed their nursing education outside of Canada [54].

The various entities of the government of Canada have been working collectively for decades on the demand to ensure that migrant health workers, including IENs arrive with permanent resident status, addressing long-held concerns and critics of Canada's approach to foreign caregivers. As part of the federal government's efforts to establish a permanent program for foreign caregivers, many IENs enter the country under this program, which would give caregivers from abroad permanent residence upon arriving in Canada, a step intended to update and replace existing programs. Most IENs from the Philippines entered Canada through the previously mentioned caregivers' programs and had been trapped in the system, facing multiple obstacles to becoming licensed as registered nurses and practicing in their specialized healthcare settings [29]. According to advocacy group interviews, migrants expressed their concerns over the status of thousands of caregivers that have faced abuse and exploitation and have been in an indeterminate state or have become undocumented over the past years, urging the government of Canada to take action in implementing a regularization program for undocumented caregivers to ensure that no one is left behind [29]. Through recent pathways, the government has also allowed caregivers to work for organizations that offer temporary or part-time care for people who are recovering from injury or illness and those who are not fully independent [29].

Although these programs give preference to applicants with comparable nursing education and credentials, the processing times may vary on the basis of each candidate's immigration pathway.

Migration of Nurses

Canada has been a county of attraction to many IENs from several countries of origin and, in most instances, from transitioning countries as a second migration. The global trends of migration have evolved with continuous modifications to the immigrant selection process, resulting in changes in the demographic and human capital characteristics of IENs. Nurses will continue to mobilize across the globe from various countries. Significant numbers of IENs come to Canada from countries such as the Philippines, India, Nigeria, the United Kingdom, the Middle East, and China. The Philippines is particularly notable as a leading source due to its strong emphasis on nursing education and English proficiency. However, many of its graduates face challenges, as do all IENs, to verify their credentials, become regulated nurses and integrate into the workplace [20].

Mobilization

IENs' inter-Canadian mobility has received limited attention, although it became crucial during the COVID-19 pandemic when urgent staffing needs arose with variations in supply and demand in various regions. During the COVID-19 pandemic, many provinces made special provisions to quickly credential nurses from other provinces, helping to address temporary surges in demand [48]. Despite the *Canadian Free Trade Agreement (CFTA),* the purpose of which is to facilitate unrestricted pan-Canadian mobility, a nurse licensed in one province cannot generally practice in another unless they meet the specific requirements of the respective nursing licensing regulatory bodies [13]. Nursing mobility is fundamental for addressing shortages, balancing workforce distribution, and guaranteeing that remote or underserved areas have access to sufficient nursing services given Canada's diverse geography and regional healthcare demands. Although nursing mobility in Canada seems to be a structured and flexible system, geographic and demographic disparities in healthcare needs, the inequitable distribution of the nursing workforce across the country, wage differences, and regional preferences remain significant challenges. With the ongoing coordination of regulatory bodies, nursing associations, and government entities, building a solid strategy for nursing mobility is promising because health care remains accessible across diverse regions.

Nursing regulators across provinces coordinate to maintain consistent standards. For example, the Canadian Council of Registered Nurse Regulators (CCRNR) works on policies that support mobility, such as aligning competency and educational requirements. Recent measures, such as expedited licensing [43], have been implemented to increase cross-Canada IEN mobility, which may ultimately impact the sustainability of the rural and remote nursing workforce (CCRNR, [12]). For the future IENs, having a streamlined national pathway for licensure process and being able to transfer their licensure across provinces and territories will allow them to pursue career opportunities that better match their skills and areas of specialization that may be either not available in their home province or very competitive in entering the job market, thereby broadening the professional experience of IENs and improving the quality of health care for Canada's diverse population. Despite the tremendous benefit of mobility, IENs still face challenges related to differences in the scope of practice, variation in wage rates, and the cost of relocation and readjustment to new communities, which sometimes make moving to rural and remote regions more difficult. Most IENs may still prefer urban locations reflecting enhanced cultural diversity and offering a greater array of family settlement supports.

As the healthcare landscape continues to evolve, Canada faces significant challenges in meeting nursing demands. Current policies hinder timely access to practice for IENs. A coordinated approach to monitoring nursing workforce needs and facilitating mobility is essential to address shortages effectively. There is a need for more proactive strategies that engage various stakeholders to ensure that the nursing workforce meets the demands of the population moving forward.

> *We need a healthy workforce to get Canadians the care they need. That starts with making sure health workers are supported so they can do what they do best: care for Canadians. This investment will help more Internationally Educated Nurses join the workforce in Canada to help our current workforce and get more nurses into our health care system even faster.*
>
> *The Honourable Mark Holland*
> *Minister of Health*

> *Internationally Educated Nurses need adequate supports to be successful as they integrate into the work environment in Canada. CASN's residency program, alongside a mentorship program, workshops and training designed specifically for IENs, will provide more targeted supports as we welcome our international nurse colleagues into the Canadian workforce.*
>
> *Dr. Leigh Chapman*
> *Chief Nursing Officer of Canada*

The Canadian Healthcare Context

The integration process of IENs, who are also new immigrants, unfamiliar with the Canadian healthcare system and face language and cultural differences, can be particularly daunting. This section includes:

1. An overview of the Canadian healthcare system
2. The levels and sectors of healthcare services available
3. The limitations of Canada's publicly funded healthcare system
4. The nursing profession and professional organizations that support nurses
5. IENs' role in the interprofessional healthcare team
6. IENs' challenges in the Canadian healthcare context

Canadian Healthcare System

Canada's universal, federally, and publicly funded healthcare system, also known as Medicare, is a source of national pride and a model of free and comprehensive health coverage. It provides relatively equitable access to primary, secondary, and tertiary care services through thirteen provincial and territorial tax-funded public insurance plans.

The Canada Health Act [10] is legislation whereby the federal government sets and administers the national standards for the healthcare system. These standards set the conditions by which thirteen distinct provinces and territories receive federal funding for the delivery of healthcare services. This model of service provision sets the context of professional regulation of healthcare providers as a provincial and territorial responsibility and not a federal one. All Canadians have health coverage regardless of their medical history and ability to pay. The Canadian Health Act also prohibits extra billing and user fees for medically necessary care delivered by enrolled physicians or hospitals [1].

There are five main principles in the Canada Health Act:

Public Administration

All administration of provincial health insurance must be carried out by a public authority on a nonprofit basis. The administration must be accountable to the province or territory; their records and accounts are subject to audits.

Comprehensiveness

All necessary health services, including hospitals (acute, rehabilitation, and community), physicians, and surgical dentists.

Universality

All insured residents are entitled to the same level of health care.

Portability

Residents who move to a different province or territory are entitled to coverage from their home province during a minimum waiting period. This also applies to residents who leave the country.

Accessibility

All insured persons have reasonable access to healthcare facilities. In addition, physicians, hospitals, and clinics must be provided reasonable compensation for their services.

While the healthcare system in Canada covers basic services, including primary care physicians and hospitals, there are additional services that are not covered. Medicare provides coverage for approximately 70 percent of Canadians' healthcare needs, and the remaining 30 percent is paid for through the private sector and/or personally. Thirty percent typically relate to services not covered or only partially covered by Medicare, such as prescription drugs, eye care only for aged and diabetic patients, medical devices, psychotherapy, physical therapy, and dentistry. Approximately 65–75 percent of Canadians have some form of supplementary health insurance; many receive it through employers, and some from social service programs for vulnerable populations, such as seniors, minors, and those with disabilities. Starting in 2024, the federal government also implemented the Canadian Dental Care Plan for adults over 65 years of age or disabled and children under 18 years of age [24]. The Canadian Government is working on comprehensive dental care for all ages. There is also a legislative framework to introduce some coverage for Pharmacare. While all provincial insurance plans cover basic services, some provinces have plans covering additional healthcare expenses.

Three Levels of Acuity of Health Care: Primary, Secondary, and Tertiary

IENs need to be familiar with the structure of the different levels of healthcare services, which are determined by the severity of the illness, so that they can access the appropriate level of care should the need arise, both as newcomers and as they relaunch their nursing career.

Three Levels of Acuity of Health Care: Primary, Secondary, and Tertiary

IENs need to be familiar with the structure of the different levels of healthcare services, which are determined by the severity of the illness, so that they can access the appropriate level of care should the need arise, both as newcomers and as they relaunch their nursing career. The levels of healthcare services in Canada are:

Primary Care: The first point of contact for health services typically provided by physicians, nurse practitioners, and other healthcare professionals. It includes the prevention, diagnosis, treatment, follow-up of health conditions, referrals to specialists, and diagnostic services.

Secondary Care: This level encompasses health services provided by a specialist or facility upon referral by a primary care physician or NP that requires more specialized knowledge, skill, or equipment.

Tertiary Care: Acute, highly specialized medical treatment/care provided mainly at hospitals [23].

Sectors of Healthcare Services

Acute care, long-term care, home/community care, and public health are the major sectors of healthcare services in Canada. Most IENs coming to Canada are familiar with the acute care and public health sectors, as they are available in most countries, but long-term care or home/community care can be very foreign to them. Most IENs, particularly those from collectivist cultures [56], look after their elderly or chronically ill in their own homes rather than in an institution.

Acute Care

Acute care is a branch of secondary health care where a patient receives active short-term treatment for a severe injury or episode of illness, an urgent medical condition, or recovery from surgery. Most acute care is provided in hospital or urgent care settings.

Long-Term Care

Long-term care comprises an array of services addressing both the long-term medical and nonmedical needs of people with a chronic illness or disability who are unable to care for themselves.

Home/Community Care

Home/community care is health care provided in a patient's residence or in a community setting to promote, maintain, or restore health or to minimize the effects of illness and disability.

Public health encompasses organized measures to prevent disease and promote health among the population, not just on an individual patients or diseases. For example, mass vaccination programs such as those for COVID-19 are conducted by public health.

Limitations of Canada's Publicly Funded Healthcare System

Increasing costs, long wait times, and multiple care providers without centralized patient centered health records (which may lead to polypharmacy and unnecessary diagnostic tests) have been cited as the current state of the Canadian healthcare system.

Costly System

While the healthcare system in Canada covers most necessary services, including primary care physicians and hospitals, there are some additional services that are not covered, including dental services for people not covered by the recently launched Canadian Dental Care Plan, optometrists, and prescription medications [23].

Private health insurance plans are generally offered as part of an employee benefit package by many employers; most of them cover medication, vision, and dental care. Alternatively, Canadians can purchase insurance packages from private insurance providers. The main reason many choose to purchase private insurance is to supplement primary health coverage. For those requiring services that may not be fully covered under provincial health insurance, such as corrective lenses, medications, or home care, a private insurance plan offsets such medical expenses. While private insurance can benefit those with certain needs, most Canadians rely exclusively on the public health system.

Duplication of Care and Diagnostic Tests

The lack of coordination and multiple disconnected health record systems managed by different levels of government contribute in part to the confusion and inaccessibility of critical health information. This may impact the delivery of timely services, resulting in unnecessary tests, extending wait times, and/or hospital stays and contributing to medication errors. Fewer than 40% of Canadians report accessing some of their health information electronically, and only 35% of physicians share patient information outside their practices. In mid-2024, the Ministry of Health introduced the *Connected Care for Canadians Act,* which outlines Canada's plan in which health information can be securely accessed by patients and shared between providers to enable timely and secure access to personal health information. The Act also requires all IT companies providing digital health services in Canada to adopt common standards and allow for protected and secure information exchange across various systems [25].

Our publicly funded healthcare system has been the subject of political controversy and debate in the country. Some question the efficiency of the current system to deliver treatments in a timely fashion and advocate the adoption of a complementary private system. Conversely, there are worries that privatization would lead to inequalities, with only wealthy individuals being able to afford certain treatments [33]. Despite the political debate, Canada boasts one of the highest life expectancies of 83.11 years and the lowest infant mortality rates of industrialized countries, which many attribute to Canada's healthcare system [36].

The Nursing Profession

Nursing is one of 30 regulated health professionals, and the responsibility of regulating all health professionals resides with each province and territory rather than nationally. All nurses, including IENs, must be registered with the regulatory body in the jurisdiction (province or territory) where they practice, and they must renew their registration annually to keep their license active.

With over 450,000 nurses, nursing is the largest group of regulated healthcare professionals in Canada with protected nursing titles include licensed practical nurses (LPNs) or registered practical nurses (RPNs) in Ontario and Quebec; registered psychiatric nurses (RPNs) in the provinces of British Columbia, Alberta, and Manitoba; and registered nurses (RNs) and nurse practitioners (NPs) for all provinces and territories. It is illegal to use these titles unless the nurse has obtained the specific category of registration from the regulatory bodies where he/she practices.

There are different educational requirements for each category of registration: LPNs/RPNs need to obtain a 2-year diploma from a community college; registered psychiatric nurses completed a 4-year baccalaureate program in psychiatric nursing from a university; RNs completed a 4-year university degree program; and NPs are RNs who are experienced nurses with additional education focusing on clinical practice for at least 2 years at the graduate level. NPs are authorized to autonomously diagnose and treat illnesses, order and interpret tests, prescribe medications, and perform medical procedures [2].

Internationally educated licensed practical nurses (LPNs and RPNs in Ontario and Quebec) made up 7% of all LPNs and 25% of the net increase in LPN supply in 2023, compared with 15% in 2022. Internationally educated registered nurses (RNs) made up 10% of all RNs and account for 68% of the net increase in RN supply (6256) in 2023, compared with 64% (3333) in 2022 and 19% in 2021. Internationally educated nurse practitioners (NPs) represent 5% of the total number of NPs in Canada and 4% of the net increase in NP supply (793) in 2023 [15–17].

To allow for better workforce planning across the nation, the federal government implemented a national nurse database—Nursys—a system allowing for better data collection and exchange about a nurse's licensing history [23].

Nursing Professional Organizations

The Canadian Nurses Association (CNA) is the national and global professional voice of Canadian nursing. It represents registered nurses, nurse practitioners, licensed and registered practical nurses, registered psychiatric nurses, and retired nurses across all provinces and territories. The CNA represents Canada at the International Council of Nurses, which is a federation of more than 130 national nurses' associations, representing more than 16 million nurses as members worldwide [18]. All provinces and territories have their own professional organizations, with the majority with representatives to the CNA.

IENs' Role in the Interprofessional Healthcare Team

Interprofessional team models are teams with different healthcare disciplines working together toward common goals to meet the needs of patients on the basis of their scope of practice and control acts. They share information to support one another's work and coordinate processes and interventions to provide services and programs. The effectiveness of teams is dependent on team members' knowledge of one another's roles and scopes of practice, mutual trust and respect among team members, commitment in building relationships, and a willingness to cooperate and collaborate.

The scope of practice of nursing may differ from that of IENs' previous practice, and the different roles of members of the interprofessional team may be foreign to IENs. IENs need to familiarize themselves with these differences to avoid practicing out of scope of their practice or being perceived negatively by practicing below their scope of practice.

Effective teams recognize the patient as the center of the team and ensure that care is respectful of, and responsive to, individual patient preferences, needs, and values. They guarantee that the patient has input and that the patients' values guide all clinical decisions. Some IENs from hierarchical and authoritative practice environments, seeing themselves as experts, may expect clients to accept a plan of care without question. IEN must adopt the patient centered care approach and integrate it into practice as part of their Canadian healthcare system acculturation process.

IENs' Challenges in the Canadian Healthcare Context

A lack of coordination among different levels of government (federal, provincial/territorial, municipal) in immigration policies (related to health and human resource needs), healthcare services and education, and inconsistent licensure requirements resulted in confusion and mismatch for internationally educated healthcare professionals [46]. Although the registered nurse registration examination in English has been standardized across the country, other than in Quebec, where passing a French examination is the expectation, national variations still exist in credential and language evaluation standards and policies for licensure. These variations lead to inconsistency, confusion, and a lack of transparency and fairness in the credentialing process for IENs, thus delaying their return to practice [50]. Rapid changes in registration requirements were prevalent during the COVID-19 pandemic and continued into the post-COVID-19 era.

Despite major progress, including partial support for dental care, since the inception of Canada's Health Act [10], Canada's health systems did not implement the full vision of the founders of the Act, which included universal publicly funded pharmacare, home care, and long-term care. The decentralized Canadian healthcare system can be confusing to IENs who are newcomers both professionally and personally. The regulation of healthcare professionals is the mandate of provinces and territories. There is not one Canadian registration for all nurses; they need to obtain registration in the province or territory where they reside. IENs can also be challenged in finding the right categories of care providers should they or their family members need health care.

IEN Profile

Canada has an active program for permanent immigration and a long history of welcoming IENs. In the last decade, there has been a dramatic increase in the number of IENs, many from developing countries, who migrated to Canada. They constitute an important share of Canada's nursing and healthcare support workforce, with those from Southeast Asia and the Philippines representing a high proportion of workers in nursing and healthcare support occupations [15, 16].

The Canadian IEN workforce is largely female, middle-aged, and racially diverse. Although males represent a higher proportion of those who immigrated since 2002, with 91% of regulated nurses being women, nursing continues to be a female-dominated profession [22].

The Philippines educate the largest proportion of IENs, making up approximately one-fifth of the Canadian supply. A shift in the country of education is notable in that the historical primary source countries for IENs are no longer westernized developed countries such as the United Kingdom or the United States, but rather a variety of developing countries throughout Africa, Asia, Europe, and the Middle East. The change in country of education is most likely the result of global migration trends, with migrants moving from developing economies to developed economies in search of well-paying jobs, professional development or career advancement opportunities, improved quality of life, and stable sociopolitical environments [14]. Canadian Institute for Health Information in its Health Workforce in Canada 2022-Quick Stats report illustrated the total number employed in nursing- and health-related occupations by country of birth or origin.
Southeast Asia: 45,940
Philippines: 44,380
Caribbean and Bermuda: 22,220
Southern Asia: 15.190
India 2,225
Haiti: 10,880

Regulated nurses are NPs, RNs, LPNs, and registered psychiatric nurses (RPNs). RPNs are regulated only in the four Western provinces (Manitoba, Saskatchewan, Alberta, and British Columbia) and Yukon. Data for Nunavut are not available. In Ontario, licensed practical nurses are referred to as registered practical nurses. LPNs are the youngest group of nurses, with an average age of approximately 41 years. The average age of RNs, NPs, and RPNs ranged from 43 to 44 years. As a group, the nursing workforce is becoming younger, with average ages among each license type decreasing slightly over the past year [54].

Licensure Process

There is currently no pan-Canadian licensure process, as health care is a provincial responsibility.

Prior to 2014, professional recertification in Canada involved nurses whose professional credentials were formally verified and assessed through the appropriate provincial or territorial nursing regulatory body. In all jurisdictions, to become eligible to take a licensure examination, nurses must provide evidence of identity, educational equivalence, previous registration as a nurse in another country (if applicable), evidence of suitability and ability to practice nursing safely, and demonstrate language competency (English and/or French). In 2014, a National Nursing Assessment Service (NNAS) was established by nursing regulatory bodies to provide a single process for IEN credentials to be verified and their education compared to Canadian nursing Entry to Practice Competencies. Serving all provinces (excluding Quebec, Yukon, Nunavut, and the Northwest Territories), NNAS issues Advisory Reports for all three nursing designations: registered nurses (RNs), licensed practical nurses (LPNs), and registered psychiatric nurses (RPNs) [41].

Recognizing that IENs were frequently taking longer than 1 year, it takes their Canadian-educated counterparts to pass the licensure examination; in June 28, 2023, NNAS introduced a new expedited credentialing service for IENS. With this new service, NNAS Advisory Reports were released within five business days of all documents being received. Those applying to Manitoba, Saskatchewan, Prince Edward Island, New Brunswick, Newfoundland and Labrador, British Columbia, and Nova Scotia are eligible for this expedited process.

During the post-COVID era, owing to the escalating need for nurses, many provinces initiated additional steps to expedite the licensure of IENs, resulting in greater recognition of international nursing education from India, Nigeria, the United States, the United Kingdom, Australia, and New Zealand. Registered nurses from these designated countries who are considered in "good standing and good character" may be eligible for registration and not need any additional requirements other than passing the national entrance examination. Nurses whose education does not meet the "international requirement" may be required by the regulatory body to take additional training, such as additional language training and testing, as well as a nursing bridging program or additional training. However, all regulators mandate a 3- to 5-year time limit for IENs to become registered, following which they may be required to complete additional remedial measures to ensure practice competency. This can include taking refresher courses, returning to their home country to engage in active practice, or other provincial-specific directives, such as Ontario's Supervised Practice Experience Partnership (SPEP) allowing IENs to gain Canadian experience while preparing for registration. Alberta also has a similar program to provide clinical experience and mentorship. If provincially required, the IEN may also be asked to take a jurisprudence examination that tests understanding of Canadian nursing guidelines, laws, and practice standards. Once all the registration requirements have been met, the regulatory body advises IEN applicants when it is time to take the nursing examination. Additionally, many provinces, through government funding, are now covering application and assessment fees for IENs.

Canadian Institute for Health Information in its *2024 Supply of internationally educated health professionals* reported on the pan-Canadian percentages of newly registered internationally educated nurses in 2022 which ranged from the low of 4% in Newfoundland, a 100% increase from 2017, to the high of 22% in Ontario, a 96% increase over 2017.

Perfecting language skills, learning the occupational-specific vocabulary used in the workplace, and understanding the scope of nursing practice in Canada have been identified as critical facilitators contributing to IENs successfully passing the licensure examination.

IENs are encouraged to begin the registration process from outside Canada through programs such as the CARE Centre for Internationally Educated Nurses' Pre and Post Arrival Supports and Services Program (PASS). The PASS program, funded by the Government of Canada, provides support to IENs while in their countries of residence and post arrival, who have been approved for immigration to Canada.

Workplace

The workforce integration of IENs in Canada consists of two significant milestones [20]:

1. Achieving professional recertification as a regulated nurse, accomplished by achieving success on a licensure examination
2. Securing employment as a regulated nurse

Once registered, IENs must search for employment. Some IENs prearrange their employment before migrating, but most wait until after they enter Canada to begin their job search. Many IENs assume that because they were admitted to Canada, a country where nurses are "needed," finding employment in their chosen area or locality will be relatively easy. However, depending on the economy and the job market, securing employment in their chosen setting or clinical area may be challenging for some IENs. Becoming acquainted with the different sectors and settings within the Canadian healthcare system and learning how to apply for jobs and to complete the interview process are strategies IENs can use to accelerate their employment. Oftentimes, IENs rely on their social network of friends and family in Canada to help them navigate the job search and hiring process.

Encouragingly, licensure processes are being streamlined, and IENs, with their global clinical experience and linguistic and cultural knowledge, are gradually becoming more fully recognized as an untapped source of nursing resources. In 2021, approximately 8.9% of the Canadian nursing workforce were IENs. Overall, nurses make up 48.2% of the Canadian healthcare workforce, with Ontario (22%) and Nova Scotia (19%) leading the country with the largest proportions of IENs in their supply of newly licensed nurses in 2022. In response to the AIP-enhanced immigration pathway, these provinces experienced some of the largest increases relative to previous years.

In 2021 (CIHI), 459,005 regulated nurses were eligible to practice in Canada. The distribution of nurses by license type is as follows:

- A total of 312,382 registered nurses (RNs) represented a growth of 2.5% from 2020.
- A total of 7,400 nurse practitioners (NPs) have grown by 10.7% since 2020, the largest increase in all nursing designations. In fact, NPs have become among the fastest growing professions in health care.
- A total of 132,886 licensed practical nurses and registered practical nurses (LPNs and RPNs) represented a growth of 1.6% from 2020.
- A total of 6,337 registered psychiatric nurses represented a growth of 3.6% from 2020.

Percentage of regulated nurses by employment setting:
A total of 54.6% worked in a hospital
A total of 13.7% worked in community health
A total of 13.6% worked in a nursing home/long-term care
7.4% worked in other employment settings

Employment status of nurses in the workforce:
A total of 60.8% of the workforce employed full-time
29.6% were employed part-time
9.5% were employed on a casual basis

Among all categories of regulated nurses, possibly reflective of rising urban diversity, the percentage working in rural/remote regions declined between 2020 and 2021.

In 2022, IENs represented an average of 12% of new nurses across provinces and territories, an inflow of over 5,000 IENs. While Canada leverages IENs to create a sufficient health workforce supply for the country and although the data look encouraging, not all landed immigrants with international nursing education are currently employed in health care. CIHI 2022 reports that only 42% of Internationally Educate Health Professionals (IEHPs) who were educated in nursing were employed as registered nurses, registered psychiatric nurses, or licensed practical nurses and that the health workforce supply is struggling to keep up with the increased demand for health services, notably caused by our aging population. This mismatch between supply and demand results in decreased access to primary care for patients.

IENs seem more likely to be hired if they participate in bridging programs, have professional experience in Canada or an equivalent healthcare setting, have strong language skills, and are willing to work in hard-to-fill sectors of the healthcare system, such as long-term care or regions of the country with vacancies, such as rural or remote areas [28]. Employers report that to be hired, IENs must have the necessary knowledge, nursing competencies, professional experience, and language skills to practice safely. On the other hand, employers need to acknowledge the bias existing in workplace culture, as evidenced by IENs reporting that they are often left afloat in a new job without an assigned preceptor and that they are assigned non nursing duties more than their non-IEN counterparts. They found that their opinions or suggestions were discounted, and some employers adopted a "our way is the right way" approach. This was compounded by the fact that IENs are frequently paid at an entry-level rate or salary despite having significant clinical experience in other countries of registration [32].

Recognizing the hiring challenges and appreciating that the skills, expertise, and experience brought to Canada by IENs were crucial in filling the nursing labor shortage across Canada and Ontario, the CARE Centre, with government funding, implemented the Workplace Integration Program. Educational sessions, equipping employers with the skills to facilitate smooth recruitment, successful integration, and sustained retention of IENs into their workforce while empowering IENs to succeed and excel in practice and the workplace, were scheduled. Delivered either face to face, hybrid, or virtually, these sessions, customized to address real organizational issues, offered both short- and long-term concrete solutions.

The Livingston PRESS framework (2020) referred to as " A Road Map for Racial Equity" speaks about unpacking systemic barriers and determining organizational commitment while offering nurse leaders a process to achieve not only racial equity but also authentic organizational diversity.

P – Problem awareness – **R** – Root cause analysis -	Do I understand what the problem is and where it comes from?
E – Empathy –	Do I care enough about the problem and the people it harms?
S – Strategic Connections – **S** - Sacrifice -	Do I know how to correct the problem and am I willing to do it?

> "Retention is the absolute priority, or this situation will worsen. Our next priority should be recruiting more nurses. We also need to ensure that nurses are not only working to their full scope of practice, but that it be expanded to increase their productivity."
>
> CNA President Sylvain Brousseau

Community

IENs are also newcomers, and as such, they need professional and social supports that are collaborative, multifaceted, and multi-organizational.

The measures of community engagement include the importance of ethnic ancestry, the importance of customs and traditions, and belonging to an ethnic group. Ethnic attachments are positively related to a sense of well-being and belonging to Canada [49].

Indicators of well-being cover the following domains:

- Work
- Housing
- Family life
- Social participation
- Leisure
- Health
- Security
- Environment
- Financial security
- Learning

Belonging refers to the sense of acceptance, connection, and inclusion that individuals feel within a group or community. Belonging impacts various aspects of an individual's life, including their mental and emotional well-being, social connections, academic performance, and overall happiness. Individuals who feel supported and understood are more resilient and can often cope more effectively with challenging situations [45].

When planning strategies to build a belonging community, remember:

- Every conversation is an opportunity to grow connections and increase the knowledge and understanding of the community. With respect to belonging, even small steps matter.
- Lead with curiosity by gathering people's perspectives instead of guessing at them helps them better understand what is needed.
- Bridges of connection and relationships are powerful tools for supporting a community's equity and inclusion work.
- Relationships with a community help assess whether changes successfully move individuals closer toward a goal of belonging.
- Every individual can help improve belonging for others and, while doing so, strengthen their own belonging, too.

The CARE Centre's PASS program provides IENs with information on how to move, live, and work in Canada. Connecting with other pre-arrival services, potential employers and settlement organizations help facilitate that sense of acceptance, connection, and inclusion. Once in Canada, the Care Centre's STARS program continues to provide holistic support to IENs. Based on a comprehensive assessment, a highly experienced team of case managers guide IENs through the regulatory and settlement processes with the goals of successful registration, sustained employment, and social integration. Services are provided in a culturally sensitive environment, respecting the uniqueness of all members. The CARE Centre case management program model, presented as Fig. 1 [19], places the IEN at the center of everything they do.

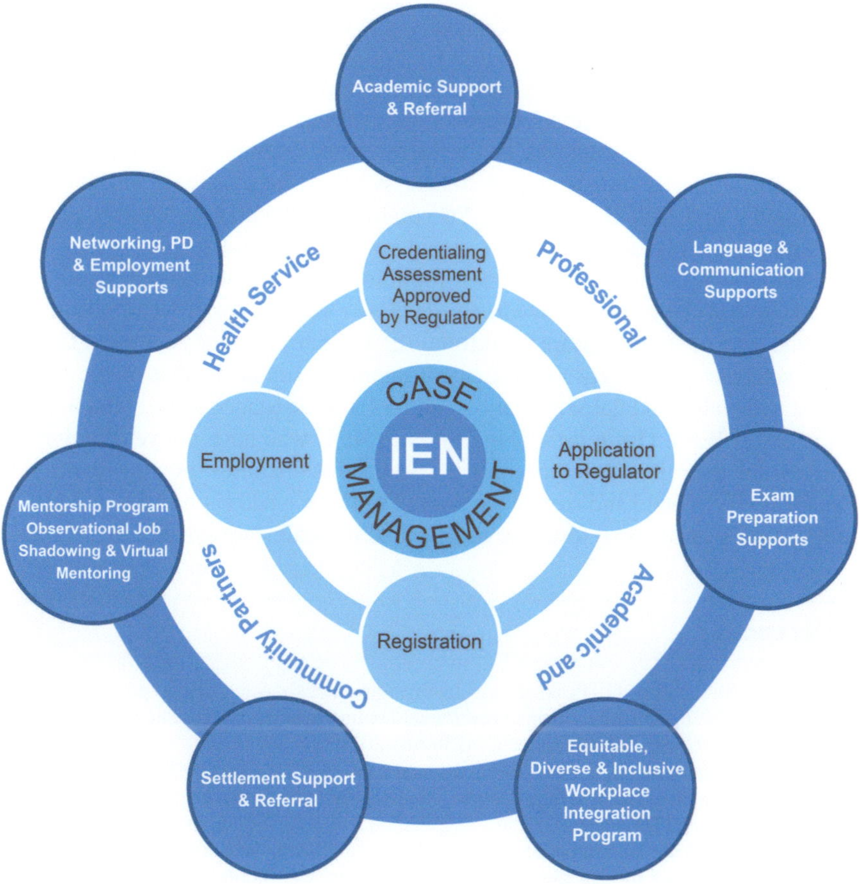

Fig. 1 CARE Centre for Internationally Educated Nurses Case Management Model [19]

"Newcomers are an integral part of our communities. Their full inclusion in our health care workforce will help us address staffing shortages, while also incorporating richly diverse voices of lived experience and better supporting other newcomers."

Alex Munter, CEO and President, CHEO N4

Conclusion

IENs will continue to migrate from a wide variety of countries throughout the world that have dissimilar nursing education and health systems. Thus, IENs are not a homogenous group, and a "one-size-fits-all" model is not effective for facilitating professional recertification, employment, and social integration in the destination country. IENs can help diversify Canada's nursing workforce to better reflect the larger Canadian population and ease the current nursing shortage. To combat the nursing shortage, the Canadian government and stakeholders (nursing leaders, academic institutions, professional organizations, and employers) have implemented multiple initiatives as solutions in the recruitment, retention, and integration of nurses, including IENs, into the healthcare system. Many of these initiatives are time-limited and lack coordination. Successful implementation requires partnerships between all levels of government and key players [6]. By simplifying immigration pathways, funding credential recognition, and offering settlement support, Canada is creating a more efficient and attractive process for IENs to become an essential part of its healthcare workforce. In addition to other countries, Canada could consider using a case management approach similar to that of the CARE Centre to develop and tailor education and forms of assistance to meet the individual needs of IENs. Using technology to reach IENs who have not yet immigrated can expedite their timely entrance into the destination countries' nursing workforce. Canada needs to build and sustain its nursing workforce and support the integration of IENs that Canada is so fortunate to have into its healthcare system.

References

1. Allin S, Marchildon G, Peckham A. International health care system profiles: Canada [Internet]. 2020. Available from: https://www.commonwealthfund.org/international-health-policy-center/countries/canada. Accessed 30 Aug 2024.
2. Almost J. Regulated nursing in Canada: the landscape in 2021. Canadian Nurses Association; 2021. Available from: https://www.cna-aiic.ca/en/nursing/regulated-nursing-in-canada. Accessed 9 July 2024.
3. Banerjee R, Reitz J, Oreopoulos P. Do large employers treat racial minorities more fairly? An analysis of Canadian field experiment data. Can Public Policy. 2018; 10.3138/cpp.2017-033. Available from: https://oreopoulos.faculty.economics.utoronto.ca/wp-content/uploads/2020/05/banerjee-et-al-do-large-employers-treat-racial-minorities-more-fairly-cpp-2018.pdf.
4. Baumann A, Crea-Arsenio M. The crisis in the nursing labour market: Canadian policy perspectives. Healthcare. 2023;11:1954. Accessed 27 June 2024. Available from: https://doi.org/10.3390/healthcare11131954.

5. Baumann A, Smith V, Crea-Arsenio M. Innovative nursing employment initiatives to strengthen and sustain the health workforce in Canada. Healthc Manage Forum. 2024;37(4):251–7. https://doi.org/10.1177/08404704241232668. Available from: https://journals.sagepub.com/doi/abs/10.1177/08404704241232668.
6. Ben-Ahmed HE, Bourgeault IL. Sustaining the Canadian nursing workforce: targeted evidence-based reactive solutions in response to the ongoing crisis. Nurs Leadersh. 2023;35(4):14–28. https://doi.org/10.12927/cjnl.2023.27076. Accessed 12 July 2024. Available from: https://www.longwoods.com/content/27076/nursing-leadership/sustaining-the-canadian-nursing-workforce-targeted-evidence-based-reactive-solutions-in-response-to.
7. Boudreau C, Rhéaume A. Impact of the work environment on nurse outcomes: a mediation analysis. West J Nurs Res. 2024;46(3):210–8. https://doi.org/10.1177/01939459241230369. Accessed 27 June 2024. Available from: https://journals.sagepub.com/doi/10.1177/01939459241230369.
8. British Columbia College of Nurses and Midwives. The pathway, partners & future opportunities. 2024. Available from: https://bccare.ca/wp-content/uploads/2024/06/12_BCCNM_IEN-Pathway.pdf. Accessed 15 July 2024.
9. Canada Health. Supporting internationally educated nurses joining the Canadian health workforce [Internet]. Government of Canada; 2024 [cited 2024 Sept 12]. Available from: https://www.canada.ca/en/health-canada/news/2024/03/supporting-internationally-educated-nurses-joining-the-canadian-health-workforce.html.
10. Canada Health Act. Canada Health Act 1985 [Internet]. Government of Canada; 1985. Available from: https://laws-lois.justice.gc.ca/PDF/C-6.pdf. Accessed 26 July 2024.
11. Canadian Association of Schools of Nursing. IEN mentorship program. 2024. Available from: https://cnei-icie.casn.ca/our-programs/residency-program/ien-mentorship-program/. Accessed 15 July 2024.
12. Canadian Council of Registered Nurse Regulators (CCRNR). Home. Available from: https://www.ccrnr.ca/.
13. Canadian Free Trade Agreement (2024)| Accord de libre-échange Canadien [Internet]. Regulatory Reconciliation and Cooperation Table (RCT); 2024. Available from: https://www.cfta-alec.ca/.
14. Canadian Institute for Health Information (CIHI). Nursing in Canada, 2018 A Lens on Supply and Workforce. Available from: https://www.cihi.ca/sites/default/files/document/regulated-nurses-2018-report-en-web.pdfNursing in Canada, 2018
15. Canadian Institute for Health Information. Health Workforce in Canada, 2022 — Quick Stats [Internet]. Ottawa, ON: CIHI; 2023a. Available from: https://www.cihi.ca/sites/default/files/document/health-workforce-quickstats-2022-data-tables-en.xlsx.
16. Canadian Institute for Health Information. Nursing in Canada [Internet]. 2023b. Available from: https://www.cihi.ca/en/search?sort_by=field_published_date&items_per_page=20&query=Internationally+educated+nurses. Accessed 26 July 2024.
17. Canadian Institute for Health Information. The state of the health workforce in Canada, 2022. Ottawa, ON: CIHI; 2022. Accessed 26 June 2024.
18. Canadian Nurses Association. Latest health workforce data confirms CNA's predictions of critical nursing shortages. 2024. Accessed 27 June 2024.
19. CARE Centre for Internationally Educated Nurses. 2024. Available from: https://care4nurses.org/.
20. Covell CL, Primeau MD, Kilpatrick K, St-Pierre I. Internationally educated nurses in Canada: predictors of workforce integration. Hum Resour Health. 2017;15(1):26. https://doi.org/10.1186/s12960-017-0201-8.
21. Dennler K. The leaky bucket: a study of immigrant retention trends in Canada. The Conference Board of Canada: Ottawa; 2023.
22. Frank K, Park J, Cyr P, Weston S, Hou F. Internationally educated health care professionals in Canada: sociodemographic characteristics and occupational distribution. Econ Soc Rep. 2023; Available from: https://www150.statcan.gc.ca/n1/pub/75-006-x/2023001/article/00004-eng.htm.

23. Government of Canada. Government of Canada announces support to improve health workforce planning for nurses, at the International Council of Nurses Congress [Internet]. 2023. Available from: https://www.canada.ca/en/health-canada/news/2023/07/government-of-canada-announces-support-to-improve-health-workforce-planning-for-nurses-at-the-international-council-of-nurses-congress.html. Accessed 30 Aug 2024.
24. Government of Canada. Immigrate through express entry. 2024a. Available from: https://www.canada.ca/en/immigration-refugees-citizenship/services/immigrate-canada/express-entry.html.
25. Government of Canada. Immigrate as a provincial nominee. 2024b. Available from: https://www.canada.ca/en/immigration-refugees-citizenship/services/immigrate-canada/provincial-nominees.html. Accessed 8 Aug 2024.
26. Health Canada. Nursing retention toolkit: improving the working lives of nurses in Canada [Internet]. 2024. Cat.: H22-4/38-2024E-PDF, ISBN: 978-0-660-70405-0, Pub.: 230773. Available from: https://www.canada.ca/content/dam/hc-sc/documents/services/health-care-system/health-human-resources/nursing-retention-toolkit-improving-working-lives-nurses/nursing-retention-toolkit-improving-working-lives-nurses.pdf. Accessed 31 July 2024.
27. Health Workforce (HWF). WHO global code of practice on the international recruitment of health personnel [Internet]. 2010. Available from: https://www.who.int/publications/i/item/wha68.32.
28. Higginbottom GMA. Experience and transitioning of internationally educated nurses (IENs) into the Canadian healthcare system: a focused ethnography. BMC Nurs. 2011;10:14. https://doi.org/10.1186/1472-6955-10-14. Available from: https://bmcnurs.biomedcentral.com/articles/10.1186/1472-6955-10-14.
29. Immigration, Refugees and Citizenship Canada. Immigrate to Canada [Internet]. Government of Canada; 2024. Available from: https://www.canada.ca/en/immigration-refugees-citizenship/services/immigrate-canada.html.
30. International Council of Nurses. ICN voices its concern about high-income countries recruiting nurses from nations that can ill-afford to lose their precious staff. 2023. Available from: https://www.icn.ch/news/icn-voices-its-concern-about-high-income-countries-recruiting-nurses-nations-can-ill-afford.
31. Lawrence K, Boyd K, Rashleigh L, DasGupta T. From recruitment to retention: evaluating the experiences of internationally educated nurses in the supervised practice experience partnership. Nurs Leadersh. 2023;35(4):30–41. https://doi.org/10.12927/cjnl.2023.27075.
32. Lee R, Wojtiuk R. Transition of internationally educated nurses into practice: what we need to do to evolve as an inclusive profession over the next decade. Nurs Leadersh (Tor Ont). 2021;34(4):50–60. https://doi.org/10.12927/cjnl.2021.26384.
33. Lee SK, Rowe BH, Mahl SK. Increased private healthcare for Canada: is that the right solution? Healthc Policy. 2021;16(3):30–42. https://doi.org/10.12927/hcpol.2021.26435.
34. Lone W. Canada's surging cost of living fuels reverse immigration. 2023. Available from: https://www.reuters.com/world/americas/canadas-surging-cost-living-fuels-reverse-immigration-2023-12-09/. Accessed 6 July 2024.
35. Lum L, Dowedoff P, Englander K. Internationally educated nurses' reflections on nursing communication in Canada. Int Nurs Rev. 2016;63:344–51. https://doi.org/10.5176/2010-48042.2.78.
36. Macrotrends. Canada life expectancy 1950–2024 [Internet]. 2024. Available from: https://www.macrotrends.net/countries/CAN/canada/life-expectancy. Accessed 7 Aug 2024.
37. McCallum AM, Vandenberg H, Penz KL. Can J Nurs Res. 2024;56(2):134–50. https://doi.org/10.1177/08445621231204962. Accessed 28 June 2024
38. McGillis Hall L, Jones C, Lalonde M, Strudwick G, McDonald B. Not very welcoming: a survey of internationally educated nurses employed in Canada. GSTF J Nurs Health Care. 2015;2(2):60–5. https://doi.org/10.5176/2010-4804_2.2.78.
39. Miller Hynds O. How changing the narrative in nursing schools could be an important step towards decolonizing the workplace. Can Nurse. 2024. Available from: https://www.canadian-

nurse.com/blogs/cn-content/2024/02/26/changing-the-narrative-in-nursing-schools. Accessed 6 July 2024.
40. Miller M. 2023 annual report to Parliament on immigration. Ottawa: Immigration, Refugees and Citizenship Canada; 2023. Available from: https://www.canada.ca/content/dam/ircc/documents/pdf/english/corporate/reports-statistics/evaluations/report-immigration-refugees-citizenship-2023-en.pdf. Accessed 28 June 2024.
41. National Newcomer Navigation Network (N4). Pathway to licensure for IENs – N4 – National Newcomer Navigation Network. Available from: https://www.newcomernavigation.ca/.
42. Nova Scotia College of Nursing. Direct international registration and licensing (DIRL) project evaluation report (interim). Halifax: NSCN; 2024. Available from: https://www.nscn.ca.
43. National Nursing Assessment Service. (2024). Annual report 2023/24: Removing barriers, creating results. https://www.nnas.ca
44. OECD iLibrary. Recent trends in international migration of doctors, nurses, and medical students. 2019. Available from: https://www.oecd-ilibrary.org/social-issues-migration-health/recent-trends-in-international-migration-of-doctors-nurses-and-medical-students_5571ef48-en.
45. Painter CV. Sense of belonging: literature review. Citizenship and Immigration Canada; 2013. Available from:https://www.canada.ca/en/immigration-refugees-citizenship/corporate/reports-statistics/research/sense-belonging-literature-review.html.
46. Paul R, Martimianakis MT, Johnstone J, McNaughton N, Austin Z. Internationally educated health professionals in Canada: navigating three policy subsystems along the pathway to practice. Acad Med. 2017;92(5):635–40. https://doi.org/10.1097/ACM.0000000000001331.
47. Pung LX, Goh YS. Challenges faced by international nurses when migrating: an integrative literature review. Int Nurs Rev. 2017;64(1):146–65. https://doi.org/10.1111/inr.12306.
48. Statistics Canada. Profile of immigrants in nursing and health care support occupations [Internet]. Available from: https://www150.statcan.gc.ca/n1/pub/75-006-x/2021001/article/00004-eng.htm. Accessed 7 Nov 2023.
49. Sarason SB. The psychological sense of community: prospects for a community psychology. San Francisco: Jossey-Bass; 1974. Available from:https://www.scirp.org/reference/references papers?referenceid=2080506.
50. Walton-Roberts M, Hennebry J, Guo J, Williams K. Immigration policy changes and entry to practice routes for internationally educated nurses (IENs). Scholars Commons Wilfrid Laurier University, International Migration Research Centre (IMRC) [Internet]. 2014. Available from: https://books-scholarsportal-info.libaccess.lib.mcmaster.ca/uri/ebooks/ebooks0/gibson_cppc-chrc/2015-07-31/1/11048791.
51. Salami B, Meherali S, Covell CL. Downward occupational mobility of baccalaureate-prepared, internationally educated nurses to licensed practical nurses. Int Nurs Rev. 2018;65(2):173–81. https://doi.org/10.1111/inr.12400.
52. Statistics Canada. Table 14-10-0412-01 Employees working overtime (weekly) by occupation, annual. 2024a. 10.25318/1410041201-eng. Accessed 28 June 2024.
53. Statistics Canada. The daily — Population projections: Canada, provinces and territories, 2023 to 2073. 2024b. Available from: https://www150.statcan.gc.ca/n1/daily-quotidien/2024/. Accessed 3 July 2024.
54. Statistics Canada. Focus on geography series, 2021 Census of population. 2022. Available from: https://www12.statcan.gc.ca/census-recensement/2021/as-sa/fogs-spg/page.cfm?lang=E&topic=9&dguid=2021A000011124. Accessed 3 July 2024.
55. Statistics Canada. Projections of the diversity of the Canadian population, 2006–2031. 2010. https://doi.org/10.25318/91-551-x2010001. Accessed 27 June 2024.
56. Triandis HC. Individualism and collectivism. Boulder: Westview Press; 1995.
57. Turcotte M, Savage K. The contribution of immigrants and population groups designated as visible minorities to nurse aide, orderly, and patient service associate occupations. Statistics Canada; 2020. Available from: https://www150.statcan.gc.ca/n1/en/pub/45-28-0001/2020001/article/00036-eng.pdf. Accessed 10 July 2024.

58. World Education Services. Summary of recent provincial initiatives supporting internationally educated health professionals (IEHPs). 2023. Available from: https://i5d8m7g6.rocketcdn.me/wp-content/uploads/2023/02/WES-Scan-of-Provincial-IEHP-Initiatives-January-2023.pdf. Accessed 12 July 2024.

The United States of America: The USA and the Global Attraction for Nurses

Vanessa Teed and Gillian Adynski

The United States, like the rest of the world, has faced nursing shortages for decades, forcing it to rely heavily on the importing of educated nurses from other countries. Nursing shortages in the United States date back to World War II, after a period of rapid growth of inpatient hospital care in the early twentieth century created more demand than supply for nurses [1]. In the late twentieth century, the opportunity for women outside of nursing, teaching, and historically female-dominated professions increased. While these advancements were good for women's rights and autonomy, the shift of women away from nursing increased the nursing shortage further [41]. This shortage has persisted consistently throughout the early twenty-first century. There was a small increase in nurses during the 2007 and 2008 recession, causing nurses to return to the bedside to seek steady sources of income [68]; however, the shortage returned soon after. The coronavirus disease 2019 (COVID-19) pandemic hit the USA in the spring of 2020, exacerbating the existing nursing shortage [60]. Today, the number of registered nurses has increased; however, it is not enough to keep up with the rising need for nurses driven by an aging baby boomer population, growing demands, and the impact of various social determinants of health [61]. Furthermore, a fifth of US nurses are expected to retire within the following 5 years [61].

To meet the demand for nurses in the USA, a market emerged for recruiting nurses from other nations and territories around the world. Staffing agencies for recruitment

Following the completion of this chapter CGFNS International has been rebranded as TruMerit™.

V. Teed (✉)
Los Angeles, CA, USA
e-mail: vanessa@vanteedconsulting.com; http://linkedin.com/in/vanessateed

G. Adynski
Duke University School of Nursing, Durham, NC, USA
e-mail: gillian.adynski@duke.edu; http://linkedin.com/in/gill-adynski-phd-rn-56ba4017b

R. El Moubadder et al. (eds.), *Globalization and Integration of Internationally Educated Nurses: A Comprehensive Analysis*,
https://doi.org/10.1007/978-3-032-01106-0_2

emerged [63]; the USA has altered laws on immigration processes to facilitate nurse immigration [29], and even, in some cases, implemented special programs and orientations to help these nurses adjust to the hospital workplace and US culture [63]. While the exact numbers can be difficult to calculate, one report states that 13% of the US population is immigrants, with the proportion even higher at 15% of the nursing workforce [34]. Internationally educated nurses (IENs) are more likely than their US-educated counterparts to hold jobs in clinical nursing and take on second jobs in nursing [33], therefore potentially directly addressing the clinical shortage of nurses.

The immigration of nurses to the USA has been a persistent tool in US policy at the organizational to national level to address nursing needs. Nurses who wish to work in the USA must take and pass the National Council Licensure Examination for Registered Nurses (NCLEX-RN®). In 2005, for the first time, IENs were able to take this exam overseas, leading to an increase in IENs choosing to migrate to the USA [21]. During this time, formal US-based firms for international recruitment began to increase [21, 57]. After the 2008 economic crisis, there was a brief decrease in IENs immigrating to the USA since many nursing positions were filled by US-educated nurses [67]. However, from 2014 to 2020, there was an increase in IEN applications to the USA again [28, 62]. In 2015, Canada, a major US sending country, implemented the NCLEX-RN® as the exam for all graduating baccalaureate nurses, further facilitating easy immigration of Canadian nurses into the USA. The COVID-19 pandemic of 2020–2022 has exacerbated the nursing shortage [60], and while nurses briefly faced issues migrating to the USA due to closure of the border during early pandemic, it is expected that the USA will rely heavily on IENs in coming years to make up for this anticipated shortage [17].

IENs are critical to the US nursing workforce beyond just meeting nursing shortages. The USA is a diverse country, with 13% made up of immigrants [34]. It also holds great racial and ethnic diversity, with 13.7% of Americans identifying as Black/African, 19.5% as Latino/Hispanic, 6.4% as Asian, and 1.3% as American Indian or Alaskan Native [76]. While US-educated nurses are getting increasingly diverse, they still do not match population-level statistics with 6.7% identifying as Black/African and only 5.6% identifying as Latino/Hispanic [61]. Nurses need to be able to build trust with their clients and understand the cultural needs of the communities they serve. The USA has faced many health disparities by race, ethnicity, and immigrant status for many decades [52], with worse outcomes in tobacco use, mental health, some cancers, cardiovascular disease, and more. The COVID-19 pandemic highlighted and brought to national attention health disparities as it disproportionately affected disadvantaged groups [35]. The National Academy of Medicine report *The Future of Nursing 2020–2030: Charting a Path to Achieve Health Equity* calls for making diversity in the nursing profession a priority to improve health equity for all Americans [81]. Nurses who represent the clients they serve can provide culturally competent care and build better trust [61, 81]. Furthermore, at the academic level, diversity in nursing faculty brings different research perspectives, pedagogies, and backgrounds that strengthen research for diverse ethnic, racial, religious, and social groups [2]. This highlights that nurse migrants strengthen and diversify the skills of the US nursing workforce, desperately needed to address health equity within this country that faces large health disparities.

The top sending countries include the Philippines (33%), India (6%), Jamaica (5%), Canada (4%), and Nigeria (4%) [34]. The World Health Organization (WHO) created a safeguard list of 55 countries that the USA and other key receiving countries should avoid recruiting from. This list includes Nigeria, which is amongst the top sending countries to the USA [85]. In addition to the top five countries mentioned above, the USA does recruit from many other countries on the list [85].

Internationally educated nurses face many challenges in their process of migration. At national levels, India, the Philippines, South Africa, and Zimbabwe have advocated against this formal and heavy recruitment as it leads to "brain drain" or the loss of highly educated individuals from their own workforces, needed to care for their own populations [41]. At the individual level, nurses face difficulties acquiring visas [63], presence of predatory staffing agencies [69], high contract breach fees [69], and agencies withholding legal documents such as green cards (legal permanent residency cards in the USA) or passports [63]. These breach fees and withholding of legal documents can force nurses to stay in unfavorable employment situations. Upon starting work, nurses face poor orientations, language barriers, and racial and ethnic discrimination at work [28]. In addition, their licenses may not be recognized, causing them to work as unlicensed personnel [28]. These IENs were also disproportionately on the front lines of the COVID-19 pandemic [17]. During the COVID-19 pandemic, Filipino American nurses have had disproportionately high levels of pandemic-related deaths compared to the rest of the nursing population [35].

To address these multitudes of challenges, the WHO created the *Global Code of Practice on the International Recruitment of Health Personnel* [84], which stipulates that the rights of migrant and domestic nurses must be equal, and that recruitment practices must be done ethically, acknowledging both the rights of the individual migrants and their source countries. The remainder of this chapter will outline the immigration and licensing process of migrant nurses into the US workforce, the US healthcare context that creates a dependency and difficulty of experience of IENs, and the integration of the IENs into the US workforce. The chapter will conclude with recommendations to ensure best ethical practices when it comes to recruiting IENs and integrating them successfully into the US workforce.

Immigration

Recruitment and Privatization of the Nurse Recruitment Industry

Welcome to the USA! The USA is home to a thriving private industry, especially in the competitive and lucrative nurse recruiting and staffing market. This competition has fueled the migration of nurses to the USA and spurred rapid industry growth. Addressing the shortage of nurses in the USA has been dependent on the recruitment of nurses from countries outside of the USA for decades [1, 17], leading to the substantial growth of the healthcare staffing industry, which is now valued at billions of dollars.

In a February 2025 interview, John Nurthen, a recognized industry expert and Executive Director of Global Research at Staffing Industry Analysts (SIA), shared his perspective on current trends in the international nursing industry. He said that, as of 2024, the value of the U.S. staffing industry was $189 billion, with healthcare staffing accounting for $46.2 billion, or 24% of the total. In comparison, the global staffing industry, which includes various sectors, was valued at approximately $621 billion. Of the overall global market, the global healthcare staffing sector represents 11%. This means, Healthcare staffing accounts for a larger portion of the U.S. staffing market compared to the global market, affirming the important role of the United States in the global industry. According to Nurthen, "The U.S. nurse staffing industry is expected to continue its growth due to demographic trends and the introduction of innovations and efficiencies." (J. Nurthen, personal communication, February 14, 2025).

A career in US nurse staffing or a nursing career in healthcare offers significant financial and professional growth opportunities for recruiters and nurses alike. Driven by financial incentives, the recruitment and staffing industry plays a pivotal role in the success of the US healthcare system as a whole and the nurse migration process itself. Agencies in the USA that assist with staffing can excel in businesses by efficiently filling nurse vacancies at the national and local levels, leading to better patient outcomes and highlighting the private sector's positive impact and its stakeholders' importance.

To understand the US market, it is important to comprehend the employment and nurse recruitment options. When it comes to employment, there are two methods: direct hire and agency hire [63]. A direct hire occurs when an independent healthcare partner directly employs the nurse and independently recruits and sponsors the migration journey, while an agency hire happens when the nurse becomes an employee of the staffing firm; travel nursing roles are a good example of an agency hire. A travel nurse is preapproved to work in various locations while the travel agency itself is their employer, not each hospital. Regarding recruiting models, there are three: direct hiring, placement firms, and staffing firms. Due to the private nature of the business, each model and each company offers different services, compensation, sponsorship, and benefits [9].

Despite the USA already having 5.75 million active nursing licenses [50], as more nurses leave the bedside prematurely or retire, domestic staffing agencies compete for a shrinking pool of nurses, sometimes recruiting from neighboring hospital systems and even from their clients without their knowledge. The current system perpetuates a cycle of short-term "staffing solutions" within the staffing industry, creating a self-reinforcing pattern. Smaller healthcare providers cannot compete with the generous salaries and appealing benefits staffing agencies offer.

The industry is seeing "an unprecedented number of nurses leaving the profession," stated Viki Good, an executive director of nurses, in an article interview by Southwick [66]. Nurses still working in hospitals and caring for patients have said they have been overworked and understaffed. Some say they do not feel safe because they do not have enough nurses and are managing too many patients. What went from we need nurses, to nurses leaving, to where are the nurses? Unhealthy trends that undermine a sustainable nursing workforce in the USA include relying on a dwindling pool of nurses, unoriginal recruiting campaigns, and clinging to outdated recruiting, hiring, and onboarding procedures. These practices act as barriers, pushing domestically trained nurses away instead of drawing them in. For example, inflexible 12-hour work schedules, unsafe work environments, inadequate accommodations for nurses with disabilities, a lack of childcare support, a reluctance to retrain nurses who have been away from the bedside for over a year, a failure to recruit more men into the workforce, and insufficient efforts to enhance educational partnerships with local high schools or trade schools are all pressing issues not only in the USA and Canada, but also globally.

By emphasizing the unique advantages of a career in nursing, such as the ability to make a meaningful difference in the lives of patients, competitive pay, and the opportunity to work in a variety of healthcare settings, more diverse individuals may be encouraged to pursue this rewarding career. It is time to take a step back and scrutinize the situation. What new and innovative approaches can we adopt to tackle these challenges head-on within the USA and decrease the reliance on IENs to avoid over-recruiting from the safeguard list?

The Business of Nurses

Immigration and emigration are natural and continuously occurring to and from various countries. However, in recent years, the International Council of Nurses [38] report *Reporting Round: Global Code for the Recruitment of International Health Personnel* has identified a clear upward trend showing that high-income countries such as the USA are relying more and more on IENs. There are two types of nursing migration: passive and active. Passive migration occurs when a nurse decides to move to live and work in a country other than their birth country [42]. This decision is based on personal factors such as individual preferences, desire for career growth, or family-influenced considerations. Active migration occurs when nurses are recruited and hired to work in other countries. This is driven by the fact that wealthier nations may prioritize addressing their own nursing shortages, potentially to the detriment of less economically advantaged countries [38].

The industry's profitability and the presence of multiple agencies have led to a surge in startups aiming to provide international nurse recruitment services. This surge has resulted in a continuous influx of new market participants ready and eager to make money quickly. The nurse recruitment industry is more than just a business; it is a vital component of the healthcare system, emphasizing the significance of the private sector and stakeholders. The international nurse recruiting industry plays a crucial role in nurse migration's success and positively impacts the global staffing market, livelihoods, access to patient care, patient outcomes in the USA, and the

US-based economy. The positive long-term impact on the sending country also benefits the nurses' local economy and family in the long term [8].

However, nursing is a business. In economic terms, nursing is sometimes framed as "human capital," a workforce of highly skilled professionals whose value is essential to healthcare delivery. Yet, this framing can leave the international nursing industry vulnerable to under-regulation and exploitation. The World Health Organization [85] has identified 55 countries with low health workforce densities that are vulnerable to over-recruitment by high-resource countries. They have advised key receiving countries to refrain from recruiting healthcare professionals from these nations. An unregulated industry poses a significant risk as it exposes nurses who are eager to emigrate from their home countries due to socioeconomic and political instability, or professional limitations, to exploitation. These individuals are vulnerable and susceptible to recruitment agencies that specifically target them in low- to middle-income and at-risk countries. It is challenging to distinguish between new-to-the-industry startups that are ignorant of WHO recommendations and those that simply do not care.

Active recruiting campaigns target accessible online professional and social platforms. This constant presence of marketing campaigns and customizable social media algorithms is designed to capture the attention of nurses already considering a career in another country. It further influences nurses ready to start the process of obtaining a US nursing license and eventually immigrating to the USA. The effectiveness and precision with which agencies can reach a broad audience of nurses globally have provided a tangible solution to the growing demand for nurses in the USA. As a result, both prospective employers and IENs rely on and look to recruiters to facilitate migration to the USA. This situation persists despite the risks. Employers face significant risks and substantial fees associated with hiring an IEN nurse through an agency as well as risks to the individual IEN, including unplanned recruitment and immigration.

The process of recruiting and employing, licensing, and immigrating a nurse is expensive and time-consuming. For new firms entering this market, it is crucial to understand the financial risks and requirements for sponsoring an internationally educated nurse (IEN). Despite the risks, the financial cost of sponsoring a nurse is outweighed by the potential value of a US-based employment contract, indicating substantial return on investment and the lucrative nature of the industry. Some contracts can be worth millions of dollars for a 2–5-year commitment per nurse, while the industry average for an IEN employment contract is 3 years or less. The determination of contract lengths is a complex process, heavily influenced by visa terms and employment agreements. However, exceeding 3 years can be considered unethical, further necessitating regulation (Álvarez, Bakhshi, & Maiyer, personal communication, September 8, 2024).

Ethical Recruitment and Call for Regulation

In 2008, the Alliance for Ethical International Recruitment Practices was established to regulate and ensure accountability in the USA and worldwide (Álvarez, Bakhshi, & Maiyer, personal communication, September 8, 2024). There is a growing push for ethical recruitment practices in healthcare, including developing a Health Care Code by the Alliance for Ethical International Recruitment Practices, a division of CGFNS International, previously known as the Commission on Graduates of Foreign Nursing Schools (CGFNS). This code aims to prevent predatory recruitment, high contract breach fees, and inadequate orientation of IENs into the US workforce [69].

In a study conducted by CGFNS International in 2023, over 50% of the survey respondents reported using a recruiter to migrate to the USA [8, 16]. When nurses emigrate, they can either pay for the process themselves or receive sponsorship from their employer or an agency. It is uncommon for agency-sponsored programs to require nurses to pay out of pocket, and if the amount is substantial, it can be considered unethical. For instance, some recruitment agencies may charge nurses over $10,000 in out-of-pocket expenses to expedite the emigration process [63]. The evolving market and ongoing United States Citizenship and Immigration Services (USCIS) immigration challenges underscore the critical importance of ethical recruitment practices. This has led to a call for country leaders and nurses to work only with certified ethical recruiters to tackle nursing shortages while upholding ethical standards.

Recruitment agencies have also been critiqued for charging high contract breach fees, or fees a nurse must pay if they terminate their contract. For example, in 2010, a New York judge denied a motion by Sentosa Care to make 27 Filipino nurses pay damages of $25,000 for failing to complete 3 years of service with the agency. This case highlighted the potential financial burden on nurses if they decide to terminate their contract prematurely. In 2018, a US federal judge allowed a group of Filipino nurses to bring human trafficking claims against Sentosa Care, underscoring the legal risks for recruitment agencies in such cases [63].

A study from CGFNS International of 1017 migrant workers, 877 of whom were nurses, found that 48 (18%) reported fees under $15,000, 81 (30%) reported fees between $15,000 and $30,000, and 46 (17%) reported fees over $30,000 if they broke their contracts [63]. Other nurses who tried to leave their jobs risk losing their visa status and being accused of committing immigration fraud [63]. This is especially problematic when nurses have cited safety issues or needing to be paid what they were promised as their reasons for leaving their positions.

Policies

Nursing in the USA is a significant responsibility that demands strict adherence to the Nurse Practice Act (NPA), the Code of Ethics, and the specific scope of practice and guidelines outlined by each individual US state and national nursing organizations like the American Nurses Association (ANA). In addition, both US federal and state laws and regulations significantly affect nursing practice. Federal statutes protect patients and address patient safety issues. State laws define the nursing scope of practice and establish ethical and practice standards for all nurses living and working within state borders. In the USA, laws and regulations work to ensure patient safety, protect the public, and safeguard a nurse's license. If these laws are not adhered to at the state or federal level, the state board of nursing has the authority to investigate and discipline. Failure to adhere to constitutional, statutory, civil, and criminal laws can lead to an investigation and judgment by the US legal system. This highlights the seriousness of legal and ethical responsibilities in nursing practice [59].

It is accurate that for-profit companies are driving the migration of nurses to the USA. The established procedure for becoming a registered nurse in the USA illustrates a successful migration process. However, when, where, and how a nurse can practice within the USA is regulated at the state and federal levels. Despite the ease of recruitment and licensing, the main barrier preventing nurses from entering the country is not the nurse migration process itself but the federal rules and regulations of United States Citizenship and Immigration Services (USCIS) and the US immigration system.

While immigration to the USA is regulated at the federal level, the nurse licensing process is regulated at the state level. The chosen US state in which an IEN selects to obtain nursing licensure must match the desired location and workplace where the IEN will live and work in. Each state has its own nursing regulatory body, such as the state board of nursing, which sets qualifications, rules, expectations, and licensing requirements for nurses practicing there. Each state ensures safe, ethical, and legal nursing practice to protect the public [51].

Influential healthcare and nursing organizations, such as the American Nurses Association, the American Hospital Association (AHA), the American Organization of Nursing Leadership (AONL), and private companies, have played a significant role in addressing the healthcare worker shortage and advocating for more employment-based visas for healthcare providers. Their decisions and actions, including lobbying efforts to increase the number of visas for internationally educated nurses, directly impact the industry. Despite the USA already having 5.75 million active nursing licenses [4–6, 50], bills like the Healthcare Workforce Resilience Act continue to be introduced to address the healthcare worker shortage and reallocate unused work visas [19, 20, 29].

The immigration regulation and visa management process are under federal jurisdiction, while the nurse recruitment and staffing industry is privatized and essentially unregulated. Despite a record number of 10.9 million applications in 2023, the backlog for immigration visa interviews in non-nursing areas has decreased by 15% as of July 2024, meeting the goal set for 2023. This progress is the direct result of improvements to the internal process, additional funding from Congress, technology updates, and the implementation of timeline markers, which have reduced processing times and ensured future efficiency [79]. While this does not immediately benefit nurses currently facing backlogs, rejections, or issues related to H-1B nonimmigrant visas or retrogression in employment-based (EB-3) green cards, it is encouraging to see support from the US Congress under President Joe Biden. Proving there is potential for improvement in the US immigration system. Although nurse immigrants are facing increasing challenges in the USA, the country remains a popular destination for nurse migrants and is expected to continue as such in the years to come.

Migration

There are three key elements in the US nurse migration process: employment, licensure, and immigration. Understanding these elements will aid in comprehending the process and the relevant stakeholders. This US nurse migration process heavily depends on the interactions among immigration services, nurse licensure, and the involvement of recruiting agencies or direct-hire employers as future employers. A nurse can only enter the USA legally with an approved visa, a US nurse license, and an offer of employment. Success in nurse migration into the USA includes three key elements, each involving multiple stakeholders. Table 1 summarizes the roles of each stakeholder in the process.

Immigration: The USCIS is responsible for the immigration process, while hiring agencies, healthcare partners, and US-based employers are responsible for meeting the application requirements, such as providing a letter of employment, initiating and covering the costs of the US work authorization application, and obtaining a valid visa.

Nursing: Key stakeholders in the nursing industry include the nurse governing and regulatory bodies, such as state nursing boards, which are jurisdictional government agencies, and the National Council of State Boards of Nursing (NCSBN). These entities, along with US-based employers and private recruitment agencies, provide essential services. For example, the NCSBN offers the NCLEX-RN® exam.

Credentialing: Nurses seeking licensure and visa qualifications must engage with education and license credentialing firms like CGFNS International. These firms offer services such as foreign credential evaluation, nurse license verification, and nurse visa screening to meet licensure requirements and USCIS application requirements.

CGFNS International [15] provides academic record assessments for international students and healthcare professionals applying to schools globally, promotes ethical recruitment practices, and monitors global employment trends. Other private companies provide the same services; however, they do not have the same impact on the global market as CGFNS International, which is a public company that fiercely advocates for ethical recruitment practices and monitors global employment trends. Additionally, they are a nongovernmental organization (NGO) in Consultative Status with the United Nations Economic and Social Council [15].

Other key stakeholders include the Social Security Administration (SSA), particularly if a nurse wishes to live and work in a US state that requires a Social Security number (SSN). Additionally, there are privately held companies that

Table 1 US nurse licensing and immigration stakeholders: role in nurse migration process and stakeholder type

	Stakeholder type		
Role and responsibility in nurse migration process	Government entities, nurse regulatory and jurisdictional government agencies	Credentialing and nurse license verification	Private companies and future employers
Required for final admission into the USA	United States Citizenship and Immigration Services (USCIS)	N/A	N/A
Required for USCIS immigration process	US State Boards of Nurses in 50 states, the District of Columbia and four US territories National Council of State Boards of Nursing (NCSBN) NCLEX- RN® exam	CGFNS International or similar privately held nurse visa screening and credentialing firms	Healthcare partners and US-based employers
Required for US RN license application	US Social Security Administration (SSN card when required)	Privately held education credential evaluation and nurse license verification firms	Companies offering miscellaneous services such as language and translation, English proficiency exams, background check, fingerprinting, and miscellaneous services
Required for the nurse migration journey	Home country council of nurses/ boards of nursing (provides valid home country nurse license)	Home country academic institutions (provides valid home country education verification)	Agency hire: recruiting and staffing agencies Direct hire: US-based employers, public and privately held companies able to hire internationally educated nurses

provide miscellaneous services and partner with individual board of nursing. These services include language and translation services, English proficiency exams such as International English Language Testing System (IELTS), Test of English as a Foreign Language (TOEFL), Occupational English Test (OET), and others as background checks and fingerprinting. Additionally, there are key stakeholders in the nurses' home country. Stakeholders who aid in the migration process by facilitating the release of essential documents. Substantial contributions from all stakeholders are crucial in the licensing and immigration processes for nurses.

As of 2020, the USA was the top destination country in the world for global migration, with over 51 million international migrants coming into the USA [39].

The USA has been the leading destination country for migrants for the last 50 years, with the second-leading destination country, Germany, not having even half the migrants as the USA [39]. Individuals migrate for a variety of reasons, including work or economic opportunities, to join family, and to seek higher education [75]. They also may be trying to leave poor conditions at home, such as conflict, persecution, or environmental factors related to climate change [75]. It should be noted that many nurses may migrate for social, family, or community reasons.

Most IENs move to the USA on an employment-based (EB) visa: an EB-2 visa for those nurses with advanced nursing degrees, or an EB-3 visa for those with bachelor's or associate degrees [63]. The USA has a large amount of visa retrogression, meaning there is a larger amount of visa applications than visas available, causing a waitlist [63]. At times, no visas are available, while at other times there is a decade-long waiting period [63]. Currently, in the USA, there is a large amount of anti-immigrant rhetoric, which has directly or indirectly led to a pause in visa applications for internationally educated nurses from 2024 [55]. For example, in 2017, US President Trump's Executive Order 13769, commonly known as the "Travel Ban" or "Muslim Ban," prevented many from entering the USA. This impacted a group of Iranian-educated health professionals and nurses who wanted to immigrate to the USA but were unable to obtain visas [63]. IEN's who are citizens of Canada and Mexico may qualify for TN nonimmigrant classification permit (TN visa) also known as the United States-Mexico-Canada Agreement (USMCA), previously known as the North American Free Trade Agreement (NAFTA) (*citation: United States Citizenship and Immigration Services (2025, June 4). TN USMCA professionals. https://www.uscis.gov/working-in-the-united-states/temporary-workers/tn-usmca-professionals). US visa eligibility, requirements, processing times, rules, and regulations are subject to change. For accurate and up to date US immigration information, please refer to the official USCIS website at uscis.gov.

Unforeseen challenges in the visa process may arise due to errors in the application itself for various reasons, leading to potential application denial. When an IEN applies for any visa type, if their application is submitted incomplete or any discrepancy is found, the USCIS may deny the application or issue a request for evidence known as an "RFE" or a notice of intent to deny via mail courier or delivered electronically [77]. Under code 8 CFR 103.2, the USCIS outlines the procedures for handling visa applications and requests for evidence issues for H-1B visa types, identifying a minimum of ten reasons why a nurse may receive an RFE. Some of the most common reasons include areas of specialty, employer–employee relationship, work availability, maintenance of status, beneficiary qualifications, itinerary, and failure to pay the necessary fees [77, 78, 80].

If the resubmitted materials meet the requested evidence requirements, the USCIS will consider the application. Application denials and requests for evidence can be stressful, costly, and time-consuming. If this occurs, the employer and nurse must be considered and kept up to date. If the delay is significant, the recruiting firm and the nurse waiting may lose the job position to another nurse, jeopardizing the USCIS application. It is important not to overlook the physical and emotional toll that this process and any delays may take on the nurses and their family members eagerly waiting to immigrate. To ensure that an IEN is well-informed during their visa application journey, it is highly recommended that they obtain the most up-to-date and credible information directly from the official website, uscis.gov. This resource provides comprehensive information relating to US immigration visa types, rules, standards, and application processes [77, 78].

Mobility

The USA is a popular destination for nurses due to various career- and mobility-related factors. The USA has implemented national pathways to facilitate nursing mobility through standardized online application processes, shared services, and initiatives like the Compact Agreement. Other desired career-related factors include travel nursing roles, higher educational and advanced practice opportunities, professional development prospects, and higher pay that may not be available in an IEN's home countries.

Organizations such as NCSBN and CGFNS International play a pivotal role in nursing. NCSBN, known for its "Exams for the Real World of Nursing" [50], operates testing centers domestically and internationally for the widely accepted NCLEX-RN®. Companies like "Nursys.com," on the other hand, are responsible for verifying US nurse licenses and ensuring that nurses meet the requirements for practice. CGFNS International offers services to evaluate international education equivalency, which is particularly useful for internationally educated nurses seeking to practice in the USA.

The Nurse Licensure Compact (NLC) enables nurses to transfer licenses and practice legally across states, and its growth signifies a promising future for nursing practice. It allows nurses to hold a single-state or multistate license, granting them the privilege to practice in their home state and other compact states. Some requirements include a valid US Social Security number, English proficiency, an active and unencumbered nursing license in their home state, passing the NCLEX-RN®, graduating from a board-approved school, and other requirements if one has a criminal background. Currently, there are 42 participating jurisdictions as part of the NLC [48, 49]. As more states join the NLC, nurses can more easily move from one state to another in times of need or increased demand for nurses.

Nurses can easily move throughout the entire USA by applying for a new state license where they plan to live and work. This long-standing process known as "licensure by endorsement," is separate from the initial licensure by examination for IENs. To qualify for endorsement, a nurse must have a valid and current nurse license in another state, meet the educational and training requirements for the state where they are applying, and have passed the NCLEX-RN® [14].

Travel nursing offers a unique level of independence, flexibility, and nationwide mobility. Nurses can choose to work in any part of the USA and at their preferred times, allowing them to shape dynamic and well-compensated careers. During the COVID-19 pandemic, there was a significant increase in the demand for short-term contract nurses, especially registry and travel nurses. This sudden change resulted in a three- to fourfold increase in individual salaries, leading to what has been termed the rise of the Travel nursing industry [87]. This shift and rise of the Travel nursing industry was made possible not by business ingenuity but by the heroism and willingness of nurses to work in dire conditions, coming to the rescue of the entire nation during the darkest days of the pandemic. Despite the challenges posed by the pandemic and the salary fluctuations, the job's attractiveness and advantages remain unchanged [72]

Professional nursing organizations such as the Board of Certification for Emergency Nursing (BCEN) and the American Association of Critical-Care Nurses (AACN) offer specialty certifications and Advanced Practice Certification pathways. Most specialty nursing associations and organizations provide nurses with leadership, perioperative care, obstetrics, pediatrics, and certification opportunities. Eligibility includes work experience in the designated area, a fee, and a standardized exam. Certifications represent a commitment to practice, excellence, and expertise (BCEN, [3, 12]).

Aspiring nurses and IENs have access to various educational and professional development pathways in the USA. Aspiring nurses can pursue initial licensure through a nursing diploma, associate's and bachelor's degree programs, an RN-to-bachelor's degree program, or a dual bachelor's to master's program. In addition to a high volume of PhD degrees, nurses in the USA can seek degrees as nurse practitioners, certified registered nurse anesthetists, nursing education degrees, certified nurse specialists, and many more degrees. A limited number of countries offer some of these advanced nursing practice degrees, such as nurse practitioner and nurse anesthetist [46], making it an opportunity for advancement in nursing that nurses may not be able to find in their countries of origin or even other popular destination countries.

Furthermore, nurses have competitive pay in the USA. The average salary for nurses in the USA is $81,220 USD [26], with some states such as California, Hawaii, and Oregon offering average salaries of more than $110,000 USD [25]. Only Switzerland, Luxembourg, and Denmark pay more than the US average with $99,839 USD, $94,923 USD, and $83,888 USD, respectively [26]. All these factors are a few career-related factors that may pull nurses to migrate to the USA.

Once a nurse obtains licensure in a US state and continues to practice in that original state, they are responsible for paying licensing fees and completing continuing education hours. The requirements vary by each state's board of nursing and typically include a license renewal fee that must be paid every 2 years.

Healthcare Context

The USA experiences the worst healthcare outcomes of all high-income nations, including individuals who are more likely to die younger and from avoidable causes, the highest maternal and infant mortality, and the highest suicide rates [30]. Individuals in the USA are more likely to have multiple chronic diseases and obesity than those in other Organisation for Economic Co-operation and Development

(OECD) countries [30]. Despite these results, the USA spends more per capita on healthcare than any other high-income country [30]. Unlike many other high-income countries, the USA does not guarantee health coverage to its residents, leaving 8.6% of its population uninsured [31].

The USA stands out with its unique healthcare system, which is not universal but a business-driven and private model. This system, with its diversified healthcare industry, offers a multitude of opportunities for nurses. It is a mix of independently owned businesses, private and public, nonprofit and for-profit, and government healthcare systems and providers, all regulated at the state and federal levels. This diversity ensures that there is a niche for every nurse, catering to their unique skills and interests [71].

Health insurance coverage is part of a unique private-payer healthcare system and offers distinct advantages for nurses. Employers pay for most healthcare costs through private insurance plans in this healthcare system. This system provides advantages for nurses, including coverage under full-time or some part-time positions as part of a benefit package. However, the offerings and costs vary depending on the employer. It is important to note that coverage is only guaranteed if the nurse can afford the estimated monthly cost [73].

Those who are unable to afford healthcare either go without or may qualify for a government-sponsored plan. The 2010 Patient Protection and Affordable Care Act, a government-funded act, ensures affordable care options for lower-income individuals and those over 65 [73, 74]. Introduced by President Obama in 2010 to offset the financial burden of healthcare and address the growing percentage of Americans without health coverage, the Affordable Care Act has led to a historic advancement of health coverage and equity in the USA. Data from 2023–2024 show 45 million Americans are enrolled, an increase of 33 million since its enactment in 2014 [7]. Although these government-run programs provide healthcare coverage to those who otherwise would not have it, the system remains private.

This system provides a stable and highly desirable nursing profession within the competitive and privatized healthcare industry. With growing demand and many high-paying career opportunities in the USA, it ensures financial security and stability, making it a financially rewarding career choice for nurses [74]. With its growing demand, it offers a sense of security and confidence for nurses in the USA and those planning to migrate.

For decades, the USA has been a sought-after destination for nurses, offering high-paying jobs, an abundance of career development opportunities, and an improved quality of life within a privatized business-oriented health system. The trend of nurses moving to the USA is on the rise, with data from the CGFNS International indicating that this trend will likely continue. This data provides hope and motivation for aspiring nurses, reinforcing their decision to pursue a career in the US healthcare system for economic, familial, and professional reasons [9, 15].

Integration

Internationally Educated Nurses' Profile

Internationally educated nurses make up 15% of all registered nurses in the USA [34]. However, this data is from 2014, and it can be difficult to find more updated data in the USA. California and New York have 26% and 14% of the international nursing workforce working in each of their states, respectively [34], which of note are also some of the higher paying states for nursing wages [25, 26]. The top countries of origin are the Philippines (33%), India (6%), Jamaica (5%), Canada (4%), and Nigeria (4%) [34]. Another study put Filipino nurses in the USA as high as 40% [40]. The Filipino nurses are a sizable percentage of the total US nursing workforce. It is estimated that 100,000 Filipino nurses work in the USA, approximately 3.7% of the total US nursing workforce [40]. Of note, the Philippines, India, Jamaica, and Nigeria are considered low- or middle-income countries by the World Bank [83], highlighting how the majority of IENs come from middle- or low-income countries. Other major sending countries or territories include Hong Kong, Japan, Mexico, Puerto Rico, South Korea, the United Kingdom, and Vietnam [41].

The IEN workforce in the USA works in hospitals (67%), nursing care homes (9.5%), followed by outpatient facilities (3.3%), home health (3.8%), and physician offices (1.6%) [34]. IENs are more likely than US-educated nurses to work full-time, work in hospital settings, and provide direct patient care, and they are less likely to work in management [28]. IENs are more likely than US-educated nurses to hold a bachelor's degree [56, 58], with recent data indicating that 77% have bachelor's degrees or higher. Twenty-one percent of IENs have more than 20 years of experience [10].

Licensing

Standardized Process: Overview of US Nurse Licensing Process

The USA has established effective nurse licensing procedures. The evidence is clear: For over 100 years, the 59 Boards of Registered Nursing have consistently maintained and set standards for nurse licensure across all 50 states, the District of Columbia, and four US territories. The Boards of Nursing across the USA are jurisdictional governmental agencies and nurse regulatory boards that uphold similar standard [51]. Each board of nursing is unique; thus, each state's website and application instructions should be considered accordingly. The application process, while unique to each board of nursing, is designed to be straightforward and manageable (Fig. 1).

The licensing process for internationally educated nurses (IENs) in the USA is efficient and highly standardized across all states, with minimal variations. Nurses who have completed nursing programs in foreign countries and hold a valid nursing license from outside the USA are eligible to apply for registered nurse licensure by examination in all states. They can do this under the foreign-educated nurse or

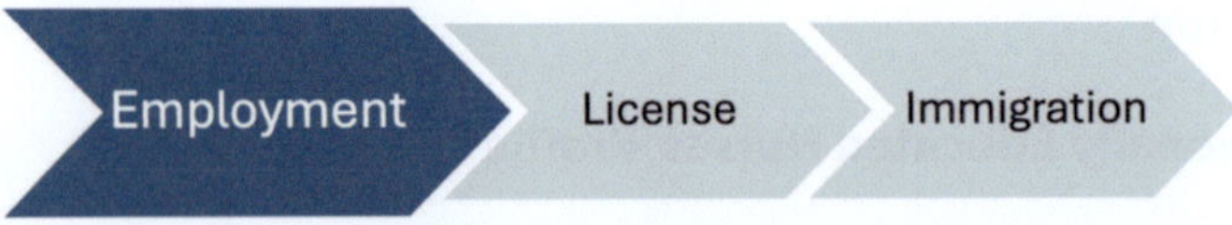

Fig. 1 Three key elements in the US nurse migration process
Definitions: 1. Employment: direct or agency hire. 2. License: any US BON application. 3. Immigration: application with the USCIS

international nurse application criteria. Each state's board of nursing website provides applications and online instructions. IEN's who have successfully passed the NCLEX-RN® and are working in a country that requires the exam for licensure and wish to obtain a license to work legally in the United States should follow the same licensing process. For example, in the state of Texas, an IEN does not need to apply for "registered nurse licensure by examination"; instead, they can apply for "Endorsement RN" (for internationally and Puerto Rico-educated nurses) [70]. In this case, IENs such as those immigrating from Canada or Australia will still need to fulfill all requirements for internationally educated and licensed nurses, but they do not need to retest if they can provide proof of having passed the NCLEX-RN® in their home country.

There are two pathways for internationally educated nurses to obtain licensure in the USA. The most common method is nurse migration, where the nurse is not physically located in the USA but plans to migrate once a nurse license, employment offer, and valid visa are obtained. The secondary pathway applies to internationally educated nurses who are already physically present in the USA for various reasons, such as residing as dependents on a family member's visa, holding a student visa, or having migrated to the USA for an alternative professional endeavor. Regardless of the chosen pathway, the process for obtaining legal US nurse licensure through examination is consistent, although the prerequisites associated with the visa category may vary.

Streamlining the US Nurse Licensing Process: Can We Learn from the USA?

The licensing process for IENs in the USA is efficient and highly standardized across all states, with minimal variations. This consistency, characterized by a clear set of licensure standards, instills confidence in internationally educated nurses regarding their ability to swiftly obtain licensure in the USA and qualify to practice as registered nurses. This standardized process allows nurse staffing and recruitment firms to streamline their operations, thereby facilitating the expedient integration of internationally educated nurses into the US market

The process for a nurse to work in the USA involves several steps: applying for a job, choosing a state for licensure, meeting the state's requirements (including document submission and exams), and paying associated fees. Nurses who have graduated from foreign nursing schools and hold a valid nursing license outside of the USA can qualify for registered nurse licensure by examination in all states, under the foreign-educated nurse (FEN) or international nurse criteria. Applications and instructions can be found online on each individual board of nursing website. It is important to pay attention to the small details. For instance, some boards of nursing like Florida, require a social security number (SSN) while others, such as the Texas Board of Nursing, do not [24, 70].

Choosing the right state to live and work in is an important decision that requires careful consideration of employment opportunities, pay, lifestyle preferences, and which board of nursing to apply to. While it is tempting to do a quick internet search on the easiest or fastest board of nursing to apply to, the application must align with the nurse's credentials, qualifications, and job prospects.

Obstacles in Obtaining a US Nurse License

When applying to US boards of nursing, internationally educated nurses may encounter challenges in states that mandate a nine-digit identifier known as a Social Security number (SSN) as part of the initial registration requirement. For instance, Florida requires an SSN, but an SSN is not required to take the NCLEX-RN®. Lawfully admitted noncitizens can apply for an SSN in the USA [64, 65]. The nurse must be physically present in the USA for more than 10 days and meet immigration and employment requirements. For instance, the Florida Board of Nursing application requires an SSN. However, an SSN is not necessary to take the NCLEX-RN®. Once a nurse obtains an SSN, they become eligible to apply for a nursing license in any US state [24].

The process of obtaining a nurse license can be expensive and time-consuming, depending on the nurse's country of origin and the difficulty of obtaining and sending required documents. The duration of the process can range from less than a month to several months, and is influenced by the ease of the process, processing times of required services, and delivery of essential documents. The time it takes to process applications can vary widely depending on the nursing board. Common reasons for these variations include document loss, rejection of documents, high volume of applications (especially around popular graduation dates such as June and December), outdated processes, delayed submission of documents from third-party vendors, and staffing shortages for application review. Given the varying fees and required services per state, effective planning and resource management are necessary for successfully navigating this process (see Fig. 2).

Community

Upon their arrival in the USA, internationally educated nurses (IENs) often face the challenge of building new communities in unfamiliar surroundings. This involves exploring how IENs form supportive networks, the key communities they become a part of, and the formal support provided by recruitment agencies.

To move internationally, most IENs end up very far from their countries of origin. They may be far from their families and miss major events such as weddings or funerals, as well as lacking the day-to-day support from their families [47]. They

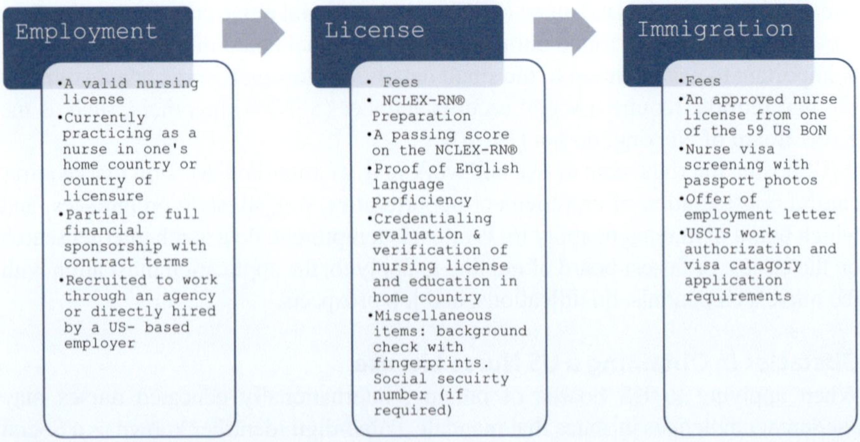

Fig. 2 Overview of US nurse licensing process

may not know anyone within the USA upon arriving, and the local US culture may be very different from their own culture. For these reasons, it is important for them to build social support quickly. Immigrants, coming from potentially very different cultures, often seek the company of those with similar beliefs, values, and backgrounds as they adapt to a new culture [32]. For internationally educated nurses (IENs), acculturation occurs at two levels. First, there is the acculturation into the host culture, and secondly, there is the need for acculturation into the work culture [47].

Integration into the host culture and social integration begin when nurses introduce and begin to gravitate toward communities like their cultures of origin. The support that immigrant nurses receive from such communities can have a significant effect on nurse retention. Research shows that immigrant nurses seek support from their families and often reside in communities with people from similar ethnicities [47]. These communities can provide social and financial support, help with setting up bank accounts, shopping, finding school for children, and finding affordable housing [32]. Research shows that socializing with other Filipinos increases the retention of Filipino immigrant nurses at their jobs [32].

Many hospitals or recruiting agencies have set up formal orientations to encourage social support systems and build communities. These orientations may include learning how to take a driver's lesson test, introductions to US weather, knowledge on US food, how to dress for different seasons, open a US bank account, get a Social Security card, and connect with other members of their community [63]. All this training can help IENs relate to other IENs but also integrate into the larger US community that they have migrated into. Studies have found that IENs who participate in formal orientation programs become more acculturated into the host cultures [23, 30, 45, 47]. These cultural orientations help decrease social isolation and prepare individuals for racism they may face [47], which in turn can increase retention and commitment to their organizations [18].

Besides these immigrant communities in the USA, migrants are also part of transnational communities. Transnational communities exist for migrants as they exist across cultures. These communities may help facilitate future nurse migration to certain locations. Additionally, nurses send money home, called remittances, which are huge drivers of home country economies. A 2023 conservative estimate from CGFNS International says that nurses send home as much as 1.6 billion USD annually [8]. These transnational communities can provide continued bidirectional social and material support for migrants in the USA and their families and friends in their home countries.

Workplace

When IENs arrive in the USA, and begin their jobs, they still face a variety of problems, not just in the first years of their work but in years to come after that. Moyce et al. [47] systematically synthesized the literature on IENs starting work abroad. This literature broke down major barriers nurses face when entering the workforce into the categories language and communication, racism, discrimination, and underutilization of skills. Strong orientation programs can help elevate these stressors and help IENs better adjust to work in their new country [63].

After starting their work as nurses, research indicates that nurses often face discrimination based on the intersections of race, ethnicity, and gender [37, 53]. The USA faces many issues with racism and discrimination existing within its society. Racism in the USA can be broken down into two types: structural racism, or law policies and institutions that provide advantages to dominant racial groups while disadvantaging others, and cultural racism, or instilled ideologies of inferiority in values, languages, imagery, or symbols internalized in individuals of that race and the society at large [35]. These and other forms of racism can lead to discrimination against groups that are minoritized within the USA [35], such as internationally educated nurses. One example of this discrimination is IENs, in general, were paid less than domestic nurses [28, 43, 82]. This can be further worsened by nurses that come from middle- and low-income countries, who receive even less pay than their high-income country nurse migrant counterparts [28, 43, 82]. Nigerian nurses in the USA reported facing racism, bullying, and inequality [37]. IENs reported experiencing discrimination from patients, patient's families, physicians, management, and other nurses [47, 53]. IENs report refusal of care from some patients due to their race or ethnicity [22, 28, 44]. This may leave nurses with feelings of isolation and lack of self-determination [60]. This discrimination at work can lead to poor patient outcomes, decreased nursing psychological well-being, turnover, or circular migration of nurses returning to their countries of origin [11, 47].

Another obstacle IENs face after arriving in the USA is that they may be put in entry-level jobs or put into settings such as long-term care, even though many IENs worked in management or teaching positions in their countries of origin [36, 47, 86]. One study of 500 hospitals in 12 countries found that 97% of IENs were asked to do clerical work, and 90% were performing non-nursing care for patients [13,

47]. IENs may need to take additional coursework upon arriving before their license is approved, if their schoolwork does not meet the criteria for evaluation for licensure [47].

However, IENs may be more likely than their US-educated counterparts to speak other languages. Globalization has caused the USA to be more linguistically diverse than ever before and having a nursing staff that is able to communicate in native languages with more patients can help provide better care [27].

These language issues may persist well beyond the first years on the job [45, 47]. This is another area where IENs may face discrimination because they may be seen as slow due to their language proficiency, leading to reduced opportunities for advancement [45, 47].

To better combat these issues of racism and language barrier, hospital or recruiting agencies can create strong policies to combat discrimination and provide language training upon arrival [60].

Past research has highlighted the benefits of strong orientation programs in helping nurses transition to working and living in a new country [32]. This orientation program can help minimize de-skilling and improve safety in the transition into their new jobs [47].

These programs have included material beyond the healthcare setting to help IENs adjust to the larger US culture such as an introduction to US banking, helping with shopping, and finding affordable housing [32].

While it is a requirement for nurses to have a job lined up prior to obtaining their visa, this job may fall through leaving a nurse without an employer after arriving in the USA. This can lead to the nurse losing their visa if it continues for too long. Finding a job is the responsibility of the recruiters; however, lack of finding a job threatens the nurse's visa status and can leave nurses in precarious financial situations [47].

Future Directions and Challenges

As we consider the future of nursing immigration to the USA, several pressing issues require immediate attention and thoughtful planning. This section's recommendations address policies at the national level, recruitment agencies, healthcare organizations, nurse regulators, and thought leaders. The complex ethical issue of global nurse migration necessitates input from all stakeholders, including sending and receiving governments and the individual rights of migrant nurses.

Nurse Thought Leaders, Regulators, and Researchers

1. Role of nursing regulation: Strong regulation supports high-quality care, nurse mobility within the USA, patient safety, and smoother workforce integration for internationally educated nurses (IENs).

2. Workforce research: Nurse researchers must investigate IEN profiles, challenges faced in the USA, and the benefits of workforce diversity, particularly in the post-COVID-19 context.
3. Recommendations:
   (a) Conduct studies on IEN integration and workforce impact.
   (b) Highlight diversity as a strength in serving diverse US populations.

US National or State Governments

1. Balancing priorities: Support individual migration rights while addressing systemic nursing shortages.
2. Recommendations:
   (a) Enforce ethical standards for recruitment agencies.
   (b) Collect and share robust data on IENs for informed policymaking.
   (c) Invest in nurse education, staffing, and leadership development.
   (d) Create international agreements with sending countries to ensure fair compensation and support.

Recruitment Agencies and Healthcare Organizations

1. *Ethical practices*: Develop standardized systems to hold agencies accountable for their practices.
2. *Data sharing*: Collect and share data on IEN demographics, visa types, and job placements to inform policy and research.
3. *Fair terms and contracts*: Educate nurses on avoiding breach fees and ensure transparent and fair contracts.
4. *Job readiness*: Guarantee job placements before migration to prevent financial and visa-related stress.
5. *Orientation programs*: Provide cultural and professional orientation for IENs, including social and family support resources.
6. *Safe work environments*: Ensure nurses work in settings with transparent pay, fair contracts, safe conditions, and adequate staffing.

In conclusion, the USA has a long history of nurse migration and remains an attractive option for internationally educated nurses (IEN). It is unlikely that nurse migration to the USA will slow down in the years ahead. Moving forward, balance is required. The USA needs to address the ongoing nursing shortage by continuing to welcome nurse migration and investing in and supporting the domestically trained nursing workforce. Strong policy decisions regarding internationally educated nurses need to be made, and the USA should ensure that the nurse recruiting process is conducted with the ethics of the individual nurses and their sending countries in mind.

The migration of nurses to the USA has resulted in many success stories, fulfilled dreams, and secured futures for the families of migrant nurses. This has been a cause for celebration and contributed to the sustainability of economies in their home countries. It has also led to a better quality of life for loved ones who stayed behind. The involvement of private businesses and the international nurse recruitment industry is essential for a healthy market, both nationally and globally. This has secured career paths, improved patient outcomes, increased access to care, and met the healthcare needs of an aging US population. This contribution should be rewarded and recognized. The USA is undoubtedly an attractive destination for nurses. However, for it to be considered ideal, sending countries should receive fair compensation, and nurses wishing to work in the USA should be treated ethically.

Additional Items

Expert Testimony

CGFNS International and the Alliance for Ethical International Recruitment Practices (Alliance).

Experts: Bakhshi, Mukul, Álvarez, Thomas, and Maiyer, Margaret

"Since 2008, the Alliance for Ethical International Recruitment Practices (Alliance) has been on the forefront of safeguarding nurses migrating to the U.S. for work—partnering with nurses' associations, labor unions, international recruitment firms, and other stakeholders to find common ground and establish a list of best practices for the ethical recruitment of foreign-educated nurses (FENs) into the U.S. The Alliance's Certification program creates stronger oversight and accountability for private recruitment firms in an industry that largely lacks government oversight, while its accessibility through open contact forms and surveys helps to elevate the voices of migrant nurses who have been harmed or taken advantage of by recruiters' unethical practices. The Alliance's work has shaped the modern recruitment landscape and brought about stronger protections for immigrant nurses, including extending open offer periods to give FENs more time to consider employment offers, increasing transparency around breach fees for employment contracts, and abolishing bad practices like charging fees for recruitment services, requiring collateral, and withholding visas and other documents.

In 2024, the United States continues to be a choice destination for nurse migrants, despite worsening visa delays and the lack of dedicated pathways for foreign-educated nurses. As the international recruitment landscape shifts due to growing demand for healthcare talent, the Alliance's work is expanding. Many new entrants to the recruitment sector ignore established best practice standards and evade repercussions for unethical recruitment practices, and the evolution of the placement model has removed layers of oversight and accountability previously enforced by the Alliance's Certification structure. In this new era of international recruitment, the Alliance seeks to expand its outreach not only to independent recruitment firms, but healthcare providers as well—ensuring that every entity involved in the recruitment and employment of foreign-educated nurses understands the vitality of transparency, fair treatment, and partnership among ethical actors. Today the Alliance continues to push for improved onboarding services for migrant nurses, including both clinical and cultural orientation, to improve transparency and clear messaging among all actors in the recruitment process, and to elevate the voices of nurse migrants in the U.S. and around the world."

(Álvarez, Bakhshi, & Maiyer, personal communication, September 8, 2024)

IEN Testimony

EB-3 Green Card: Philippines to the USA 2019 (Chester S. D. Apostol)

I am Chester Syran D. Apostol, a registered nurse from the Philippines. My journey to the USA was challenging. After 5 years of trying, I finally moved in 2019 after overcoming immigration hurdles. My nursing career began in the Philippines in 2014 and took a new turn in 2020 when I started practicing in California amidst the peak of COVID-19. Despite all I had learned about nursing and its practice in the Philippines, it was different in the USA

In the Philippines, I worked in a hospital that rarely shared reports with other facilities, and patient transfers were rare. If patients needed more treatment, we referred them to other healthcare facilities. This experience was challenging but helped me grow as a nurse. However, in the USA, it felt like I was starting from scratch. The shifts were longer, the system was different, and I had to relearn everything. To survive as a nurse in the USA, I had to program myself to forget everything I had learned and absorb everything new like a sponge. It was a challenging but rewarding process that made me reset myself and turn myself into a blank canvas again.

In April 2023, I transitioned to an RN Case Manager position, which I remain in today. The road was tough, but it taught me resilience and determination. However, I did not walk this road alone. I am grateful for the unwavering support I received from my family, friends, and colleagues. Their belief in me made a difference, motivating me to keep going as well as strive to inspire others.

H-1B Visa: Nigeria, Ongoing (R.F)

Migration to the USA is not an easy journey—it is filled with numerous challenges that require patience and perseverance. From registering with the Board of Nursing in the USA to evaluating credentials, applying for Authorization to Test (ATT), and attempting the NCLEX-RN®, each step is a test of your determination. The immigration stage is another lengthy process that demands great patience. Understanding and being prepared to face these challenges is crucial for anyone considering this journey.

I am R.F. from Nigeria, bringing over 9 years of nursing experience. I have honed my registered nurse, midwife, and public health nurse skills, graduating from the esteemed Ladoke Akintola University of Technology in Nigeria in 2011. My decision to move to the USA is about advancing my career and providing my family with the opportunity to explore and thrive in a new country.

My journey to become a nurse in the USA began in 2021. After pursuing licensure in the United Kingdom, I was fortunate to find an agency that sponsored my move to the USA. They handled my NCLEX-RN® preparation, NCLEX-RN®, CES evaluation, and US nurse licensing. In January 2023, I traveled to the Philippines to take the NCLEX-RN®. I aced the exam in one sitting. The agency even purchased my visa screen certificate and helped me secure hospital offers in three US states.

Despite the challenges of EB-3 retrogression, I have been fortunate to have unwavering support from the agency. They have filed for an H-1B visa, and though the process has been far from smooth, they have been by my side every step. Petitions were submitted, and requests for evidence (RFEs) were requested for all of them. One petition was rejected, and another was canceled on the hospital side because the position was no longer available.

Now, I find myself in a similar situation for the third time: another offer, another petition, and yet another RFE. However, with the agency's support, I am navigating the H-1B visa process, facing some challenges but remaining hopeful for a positive outcome.

Case Study

Contract Issues [54]

An NBC News article interviewed 12 immigrant health workers in 2023. These health workers were directed to work in conditions with little staff, were promised housing that was not delivered, or arrived in the USA to find they had to wait 4 months without pay for a job, despite the promises of recruitment agencies. Some nurses who were interviewed reported being paid less than their American counterparts or not being paid for overtime. Despite the working conditions being less than ideal, these individuals would have to pay tens of thousands of dollars if they left their jobs, and others were forced into arbitration or sued for more than $100,000. This article claimed that a federal court ruled in 2019 that contract penalties of more than $25,000 broke human trafficking law, as high breach fees trap nurses in their jobs due to the debt they would receive if they left.

Jeddalyn Ramos, a nurse, had signed a 3-year contract that required her to repay $16,000 if she quit or was fired early. However, she left her job in less than 2 months due to unsafe working conditions, where she was the sole nurse for up to 30 patients. Despite working extra hours without pay and facing severe penalties, she resigned, knowing it could cost her financially. After she left, the facility's owner, CommuniCare, demanded repayment, which she provided. However, the company later sued her for over $100,000, alleging breach of contract and other damages. Ramos is one of many nurses who were sued by CommuniCare for leaving their jobs before completing the conditions outlined in their employment contracts.

Acknowledgments We gratefully acknowledge the invaluable contributions of US industry experts Mukul Bakhshi, Thomas Alvarez, and Margaret Maiyer, whose insights have significantly enriched this chapter. Their expertise and commitment to ethical practices in international nurse recruitment have provided depth and clarity to our analysis, helping to ensure a comprehensive exploration of the challenges and solutions in global nurse migration.

References

1. Abdellah FG. The nursing shortage: dynamics and solutions. Reflections on a recurring theme. Nurs Clin North Am. 1990;25(3):509–16.
2. Alsulami SA, Sherwood G. The experience of culturally diverse faculty in academic environments: a multi-country scoping review. Nurse Educ Pract. 2020;44:102777. https://doi.org/10.1016/j.nepr.2020.102777.
3. American Association of Critical Care Nurses. (2024). Get certified. https://www.aacn.org/certification/get-certified..
4. American Hospital Association. (2023). HRSA awards $100M to grow the nursing workforce. Retrieved from https://www.aha.org/news/headline/2023-08-11-hrsa-awards-100m-grow-nursing-workforce..
5. American Nurses Association. (2024). 2024 ANA congressional priorities letter. Retrieved from https://www.nursingworld.org/~4918b8/globalassets/docs/ana/comment-letters/2024-ana-congressional-priorities-letter.pdf.
6. American Organization for Nursing Leadership. Bill would increase nurse faculty. AONL News; 2024. Retrieved from https://www.aonl.org/news/Bill-would-increase-nurse-faculty.
7. Assistance Secretary for Planning and Evaluation (ASPE). Health coverage under the Affordable Care Act: Current enrollment trends and state estimates [Brief]; 2024. https://aspe.hhs.gov/sites/default/files/documents/a6589500bb65294dec49d174c6ea84c1/aspe-health-coverage-under-aca.pdf.
8. Bakhshi M, Cook K, Alvarez T, Maiyer M. The economics of nurse migration: tracking the costs and contributions of immigrant nurses in the United States. CGFNS International; 2023a.
9. Bakhshi M, Álvarez TD, Cook KN, Maiyer M. CGFNS 2023 nurse migration report: navigating nursing shortages and immigration barriers. CGFNS International, Inc; 2023b.
10. Bakhshi M, Álvarez TD, Cook KN. Advancing gender equality and economic empowerment through nurse migration [Brief]. CGFNS International, Inc.; 2024. https://www.cgfns.org/wp-content/uploads/2024/03/CGFNS-Insights-Brief-March-2024.pdf.
11. Baptiste M. Workplace discrimination: An additional stressor for internationally educated nurses. Online J Issues Nurs. 2015;20(3):8.
12. Board of Certification for Emergency Nurses (BCEN). (2024). Reach your full potential with specialty nursing certification and lifelong learning. https://bcen.org/#.
13. Bruyneel L, Li B, Aiken L, Lesaffre E, Van den Heede K, Sermeus W. A multi-country perspective on nurses' tasks below their skill level: reports from domestically trained nurses and foreign trained nurses from developing countries. Int J Nurs Stud. 2013;50(2):202–9. https://doi.org/10.1016/j.ijnurstu.2012.06.013.
14. California Board of Registered Nursing. (2024). Licensure by endorsement. https://www.rn.ca.gov/applicants/lic-end.shtml.
15. CGFNS. About us; 2024. https://www.cgfns.org/about/#:~:text=The%20mission%20of%20CGFNS%20International,practice%20competency%20of%20healthcare%20professionals.
16. CGFNS Alliance for Ethical International Recruitment. Among migrating nurses: Survey shows substantially higher satisfaction rates for those who use a certified ethical recruiter [News release]; n.d. https://www.cgfns.org/among-migrating-nurses-survey-shows-substantially-higher-satisfaction-rates-for-those-who-use-a-certified-ethical-recruiter/.
17. Chan GK, Bitton JR, Allgeyer RL, Elliott D, Hudson LR, Burwell PM. The impact of COVID-19 on the nursing workforce: a national overview. Online J Issues Nurs. 2021;26(2):1–17.

18. Cheng CY, Liou SR. Intention to leave of Asian nurses in US hospitals: does cultural orientation matter? J Clin Nurs. 2011;20(13–14):2033–42. https://doi.org/10.1111/j.1365-2702.2010.03594.x.
19. Congress. H.R.6205 – Healthcare Workers Resilience Act. 118th Congress; n.d.-a. https://www.congress.gov/bill/118th-congress/house-bill/6205/text?s=2&r=1&q={"search":"healthcare+workers+resilience+act"}.
20. Congress. S.3211 – Healthcare Workers Resilience Act; n.d.-b. 118th Congress. https://www.congress.gov/bill/118th-congress/senate-bill/3211/text.
21. Cortés P, Pan J. The relative quality of foreign-educated nurses in the United States. J Hum Resour. 2015;50(4):1009–50.
22. Dicicco-Bloom B. The racial and gendered experiences of immigrant nurses from Kerala, India. J Transcult Nurs. 2004;15(1):26–33. https://doi.org/10.1177/1043659603260029.
23. Ea EE, Griffin MQ, L'Eplattenier N, Fitzpatrick JJ. Job satisfaction and acculturation among Filipino registered nurses. J Nurs Scholarsh. 2008;40(1):46–51. https://doi.org/10.1111/j.1547-5069.2007.00205.x.
24. Florida Board of Nursing (2024). Licensing and registration. https://floridasnursing.gov/licensing/.
25. Gaines K. Nurse salaries by state + the highest paying states for RNs. Nurse.org; 2024a.
26. Gaines, K. Where are the highest paid nurses? 10 Highest paying countries for nurses; 2024b.
27. Gerchow L, Burka LR, Miner S, Squires A. Language barriers between nurses and patients: a scoping review. Patient Educ Couns. 2021;104(3):534–53. https://doi.org/10.1016/j.pec.2020.09.017.
28. Ghazal LV, Ma C, Djukic M, Squires A. Transition-to-US practice experiences of internationally educated nurses: an integrative review. West J Nurs Res. 2020;42(5):373–92.
29. Goldman M. Visa freeze worsens America's nursing shortage. Axios; 2024.
30. Hagey R, Choudhry U, Guruge S, Turrittin J, Collins E, Lee R. Immigrant nurses' experience of racism. J Nurs Scholarsh. 2001;33(4):389–94. https://doi.org/10.1111/j.1547-5069.2001.00389.x.
31. Gunja MZ, Gumas ED, Williams RD II. U.S. health care from a global perspective, 2022: Accelerating spending, worsening outcomes. Commonwealth Fund. 2023. https://doi.org/10.26099/8ejy-yc74
32. Hayne AN, Gerhardt C, Davis J. Filipino nurses in the United States: recruitment, retention, occupational stress, and job satisfaction. J Transcult Nurs. 2009;20(3):313–22.
33. Health Resources and Services Administration. (2010). The registered nurse population: findings from the 2008 national sample survey of registered nurses.
34. Hohn M, Witte J, Lowry J, Fernandez-Pena JR. Immigrants in health care: keeping Americans healthy through care and innovation. Washington, DC: The Immigrant Learning Center, Inc., & The Institute for Immigration Research; 2016.
35. Hubbard SH, Gimbel J, Davood Z, Harmon M. Diversity impacts of coronavirus disease 2019. Nurs Clin North Am. 2023;58(1):59–75. https://doi.org/10.1016/j.cnur.2022.10.003.
36. Humphries N, Brugha R, McGee H. Overseas nurse recruitment: Ireland as an illustration of the dynamic nature of nurse migration. Health Policy. 2008;87(2):264–72. https://doi.org/10.1016/j.healthpol.2007.12.014.
37. Iheduru-Anderson KC, Wahi MM. Experiences of Nigerian internationally educated nurses transitioning to United States health care settings. Int J Trauma Nurs. 2018;29(6):603–10.
38. International Council of Nurses. (2024). Reporting round: Global code for the recruitment of international health personnel. https://www.icn.ch/sites/default/files/2024-08/ReportingRoundGlobalCodefortheRecruitmentofInternationalHealthPersonnel.pdf.
39. International Organization on Migration. World Migration Report Data Snapshot Top origin and destination countries. International Organization on Migration; UN Migration; 2022.
40. Jurado L-FM, Saria MG. Filipino nurses in the United States. Nurs Manage. 2018;49(3):36–41.
41. Kline DS. Push and pull factors in international nurse migration. J Nurs Scholarsh. 2003;35(2):107–11. https://doi.org/10.1111/j.1547-5069.2003.00107.x.

42. Konlan KD, Lee TW, Damiran D. The factors that are associated with nurse immigration in lower- and middle-income countries: an integrative review. Nurs Open. 2023;10(12):7454–66. https://doi.org/10.1002/nop2.2003.
43. Li H, Nie W, Li J. The benefits and caveats of international nurse migration. Int J Nurs Sci. 2014;1(3):314–7.
44. Liou SR, Cheng CY. Experiences of a Taiwanese nurse in the United States. Nurs Forum. 2011;46(2):102–9. https://doi.org/10.1111/j.1744-6198.2011.00211.x.
45. Ma AX, Griffin MT, Capitulo KL, Fitzpatrick JJ. Demands of immigration among Chinese immigrant nurses. Int J Nurs Pract. 2010;16(5):443–53. https://doi.org/10.1111/j.1440-172X.2010.01868.x.
46. Maier CB, Batenburg R, Birch S, Zander B, Elliott R, Busse R. Health workforce planning: which countries include nurse practitioners and physician assistants and to what effect? Health Policy. 2018;122(10):1085–92.
47. Moyce S, Lash R, de Leon Siantz ML. Migration experiences of foreign educated nurses: a systematic review of the literature. J Transcult Nurs. 2016;27(2):181–8. https://doi.org/10.1177/1043659615569538.
48. National Council of State Boards of Nursing (NCSBN). (2024a). Nurse Licensure Compact. https://www.nursecompact.com/how-it-works/applying-for-licensure.page#uniform-licensure-requirements.
49. National Council of State Boards of Nursing (NCSBN). (2024b). Nurse Compact. https://www.nursecompact.com/index.page#map.
50. National Council of State Boards of Nursing (NCSBN). (2024c). Number of active RN licenses by state. https://www.ncsbn.org/NND/Statistics/Aggregate-RNActiveLicensesTable.pdf.
51. National Council of State Boards of Nursing (NCSBN). (2024d). About U.S. nursing regulatory bodies. https://www.ncsbn.org/nursing-regulation/about-nursing-regulatory-bodies.page.
52. Ndugga N, Artiga S. Disparities in health and health care: 5 key questions and answers. Kaiser Family Foundation, 11; 2021.
53. Neiterman E, Bourgeault IL. The shield of professional status: Comparing internationally educated nurses' and international medical graduates' experiences of discrimination. Health. 2015;19(6):615–34.
54. Pettypiece S. Trapped at work: immigrant health care workers can face harsh working conditions and $100,000 lawsuits for quitting. NBC News; 2023.
55. Pillai D, Rae M, Artiga S. The growing role of foreign-educated nurses in U.S. hospitals and implications of visa restrictions. Kaiser Family Foundation; 2024.
56. Pink GH, Hall LM, Leatt P. Canadian-trained nurses in North Carolina. Longwoods Review. 2004;2(2):2–10.
57. Pittman P, Aiken LH, Buchan J. International migration of nurses: introduction. Health Serv Res. 2007;42(3 Pt 2):1275–80. https://doi.org/10.1111/j.1475-6773.2007.00713.x.
58. Polsky D, Ross SJ, Brush BL, Sochalski J. Trends in characteristics and country of origin among foreign-trained nurses in the United States, 1990 and 2000. American Journal of Public Health. 2007;97(5):895–9.
59. Potter PA, Perry AG, Stockert PA, Hall AM. Fundamentals of nursing. 11th ed. Elsevier; 2023.
60. Randall PS, De Gagne JC. Supporting self-determination among internationally educated nurses: a discussion. Contemp Nurse. 2023;59(6):416–21. https://doi.org/10.1080/10376178.2023.2290035.
61. Randolph A, Mattey B. Moving upstream to address health inequity: a middle school program to introduce students to a career in nursing. NASN Sch Nurse. 2023;38(1):33–9. https://doi.org/10.1177/1942602x221133125.
62. Salsberg, E. (2018). Changes in the pipeline of new NPs and RNs: implications for health care delivery and educational capacity.
63. Shaffer FA, Bakhshi MA, Farrell N, Álvarez TD. CE: Original Research: The recruitment experience of foreign-educated health professionals to the United States. Am J Nurs. 2020;120(1):28–38. https://doi.org/10.1097/01.NAJ.0000652024.67027.f7.

64. Social Security Administration. Social security numbers for noncitizens (Publication No. 05-10096). U.S. Government Printing Office; 2023. https://www.ssa.gov/pubs/EN-05-10096.pdf.
65. Social Security Administration. (n.d..). Request social security number for the first time. https://www.ssa.gov/number-card/request-number-first-time.
66. Southwick R. "Return nurses to being nurses": A call to address burnout and shortages. Chief Healthcare Executive; 2022. https://www.chiefhealthcareexecutive.com/view/-return-nurses-to-being-nurses-a-call-to-address-burnout-and-shortages.
67. Squires A, Ojemeni MT, Jones S. Exploring longitudinal shifts in international nurse migration to the United States between 2003 and 2013 through a random effects panel data analysis. Hum Resour Health. 2016;14(1):21.
68. Staiger DO, Auerbach DI, Buerhaus PI. Registered nurse labor supply and the recession--are we in a bubble? N Engl J Med. 2012;366(16):1463–5. https://doi.org/10.1056/NEJMp1200641.
69. Stievano A, Bakhshi M, Shaffer FA, Hamilton D. Ethical challenges and nursing recruitment during COVID-19. Nurs Ethics. 2021;28(1):6–8. https://doi.org/10.1177/0969733021989180.
70. Texas Board of Nursing. (2013). Licensure – Examination information. https://www.bon.texas.gov/licensure_examination.asp.html.
71. Tikkanen R, Osborn R, Mossialos E, Djordjevic A, Wharton GA. International health care system profiles: United States. The Commonwealth Fund; 2020. https://www.commonwealthfund.org/international-health-policy-center/countries/united-states.
72. U.S. Bureau of Labor Statistics. (2024). Registered nurses: Occupational outlook handbook. https://www.bls.gov/ooh/healthcare/registered-nurses.htm.
73. U.S. Department of Health and Human Services. About the ACA. HHS.gov; 2022. https://www.hhs.gov/healthcare/about-the-aca/index.html.
74. U.S. Department of Health and Human Services. (2024). Affordable Care Act (ACA) anniversary. https://www.hhs.gov/healthcare/about-the-aca/anniversary/index.html.
75. United Nations. International Migration. United Nations; 2023.
76. United States Census Bureau. (2023). United States Census Bureau; Quick Facts
77. United States Citizenship and Immigration Services. (2018). Understanding requests for evidence (RFEs): a breakdown of why RFEs were issued for H-1B petitions in fiscal year 2018. https://www.uscis.gov/sites/default/files/document/data/understanding-requests-for-evidence-h-1b-petitions-in-fiscal-year-2018.pdf.
78. United States Citizenship and Immigration Services. (2023). Permanent workers. https://www.uscis.gov/working-in-the-united-states/permanent-workers.
79. United States Citizenship and Immigration Services. (2024a). Completing an unprecedented 10 million immigration cases in fiscal year 2023, USCIS reduced its backlog for the first time in over a decade [News release]. https://www.uscis.gov/EOY2023.
80. United States Citizenship and Immigration Services. (2024b). H-1B cap season. https://www.uscis.gov/working-in-the-united-states/temporary-workers/h-1b-specialty-occupations-and-fashion-models/h-1b-cap-season.
81. Wakefield M, Williams DR, Le Menestrel S. The future of nursing 2020–2030: charting a path to achieve health equity. National Academy of Sciences; 2021.
82. Walani SR. Global migration of internationally educated nurses: experiences of employment discrimination. Int J Afr Nurs Sci. 2015;3:65–70.
83. World Bank. World Bank country and lending groups. World Bank; 2024.
84. World Health Organization. (2010). User's guide to the WHO global code of practice on the international recruitment of health personnel.
85. World Health Organization. WHO health workforce support and safeguards list 2023. Geneva: World Health Organization; 2023. License: CC BY-NC-SA 3.0 IGO.
86. Xiao LD, Willis E, Jeffers L. Factors affecting the integration of immigrant nurses into the nursing workforce: a double hermeneutic study. Int J Nurs Stud. 2014;51(4):640–53. https://doi.org/10.1016/j.ijnurstu.2013.08.005.
87. Yang YT, Mason DJ. COVID-19's impact on nursing shortages, the rise of travel nurses, and price gouging. Health Affairs Forefront; 2022. https://doi.org/10.1377/forefront.20220125.695159.

Strategic Measures in Recruiting and Integrating Culturally and Linguistically Diverse Nurses to Finnish Healthcare Context

Suleiman Kamau, Marco Tomietto, Floro Cubelo, and Kristina Mikkonen

Global Nursing Shortage and the Finnish Healthcare Context

Globally, nursing workforce demand is expected to be dire in the coming years. The International Council of Nurses (ICN) projects that, by the year 2030, the global nursing workforce will require 13 million nurses to meet care demands (ICN [15]). In Europe, healthcare contexts are facing various healthcare challenges that include nursing shortage, low recruitment, attrition, lowered attractiveness of the nursing

S. Kamau (✉)
Research Unit of Health Sciences and Technology, University of Oulu, Oulu, Finland

Department of Healthcare and Social Services, JAMK University of Applied Sciences, Jyvaskyla, Finland
e-mail: kamau.mureithi@jamk.fi

M. Tomietto
Research Unit of Health Sciences and Technology, University of Oulu, Oulu, Finland

Department of Nursing, Midwifery and Healthcare, Faculty of Health and Life Sciences, Northumbria University, Newcastle, UK
e-mail: marco.tomietto@northumbria.ac.uk

F. Cubelo
Department of Nursing Science, University of Eastern Finland, Kuopio, Finland

School of Wellbeing and Culture, Healthcare Sector, Oulu University of Applied Sciences, Oulu, Finland
e-mail: floro.cubelo@oamk.fi

K. Mikkonen
Research Unit of Health Sciences and Technology, University of Oulu, Oulu, Finland

Medical Research Center Oulu, Wellbeing Services County of North Ostrobothnia, Oulu, Finland
e-mail: kristina.mikkonen@oulu.fi

R. El Moubadder et al. (eds.), *Globalization and Integration of Internationally Educated Nurses: A Comprehensive Analysis*,
https://doi.org/10.1007/978-3-032-01106-0_3

profession, and difficult access to continued career development opportunities for nurses [17].

The Finnish healthcare system is experiencing similar challenges to other global and European healthcare contexts with a rapidly ageing population coupled with nursing workforce shortages that have exacerbated post-coronavirus disease-19 (COVID-19) pandemic [24]. Past healthcare reforms in the country have been intended towards efficiency in healthcare delivery amid a shortage of both material and human resources [5]. Recent reform that came into force at the beginning of 2023 integrated health, social, and rescue service provision from municipalities and joint municipal authorities [37]. The reform helped create 23 well-being services counties that organise integrated primary and specialised care services [25]. One major challenge faced by the well-being services counties is recruiting and retaining a sufficient nursing workforce [42].

In Finland, international nurses are named as culturally and linguistically diverse (CALD) nurses due to their cultural, linguistic, and national backgrounds. The term CALD nurse has been previously found to relieve the challenge in terminology where many terms, for instance, agency nurses, overseas-qualified nurses, foreign-born nurses, migrant nurses, expatriate nurses, and internationally educated nurses, are often used [18]. This chapter, for consistency with the Finnish context, will adopt the term "CALD nurse".

Globalisation has necessitated the movement of nurses across borders, which has been crucial for healthcare contexts that cannot sustain a sufficient nursing workforce through local education. Like many other nations, Finland is experiencing increased demand and supply of CALD nurses [35]. Nurse migration to the country has evolved since the recruitment of CALD nurses has spread to regions outside the European Union (EU) ([5]; Kamau et al. [20–22]; Cubelo [9]). Nursing is peculiar in Finland's labour market since the profession is the third most popular in the country. The entire nurse population stood at 73,688 by the year 2020, and the share of CALD nurses is still small within the workforce, and it represents about 4%, of which 69% are from outside the European Union (Finnish Nurses Association n.d.).

The current nursing workforce shortage in Finland is projected to get worse [20–22]. Reasons for the nursing shortage are like those experienced in various healthcare contexts and include, among others, an ageing population and an ageing nursing workforce where, for instance, nurses aged 55 years and over account for almost 17% of the entire workforce (Finnish Nurses Association n.d.). Increased demand for care and qualified nurses who are out of practice or working part-time jobs (Finnish Nurses Association n.d.).

To meet future nursing workforce demands, the Ministry of Economic Affairs and Employment has taken action to support the recruitment of CALD nurses and facilitate their integration into society and work life [35]. It is further intended that future recruitment of CALD nurses to Finland would alleviate the existent shortages and contribute to the delivery of safe and quality care since nurses constitute the higher proportion of healthcare professionals in the healthcare system in Finland as demonstrated by the higher proportion of nurses (18.9%) compared to doctors (3.6%) per a population of 1000 [42].

Immigration, Credentialing Pathways and Reskilling of CALD Nurses in Finland

For over a decade, Finland has been actively recruiting CALD nurses from abroad to fill the shortage of nurses. Initial efforts were directed at European Union and European Economic Area (EU&EEA) countries like Estonia and Spain [56]. In recent times, however, Finland has not only recruited within the EU/EEA countries but also actively from other countries, including the Philippines ([7], [56]), while newcomers into its foreign source markets include nations such as Vietnam, India, Kenya, and Myanmar [6, 20–22]. However, upon arrival in Finland, many CALD nurses are placed into nursing or care-assistant roles rather than registered nursing (RN) positions [56]. Many employers have been placing CALD nurses into apprenticeship positions to become licensed practical nurses (LPNs), not RNs. RN licensure is unsupported and optional [56]. This contributes to deskilling CALD nurses, meaning that their expertise is underutilised in Finland, resulting in downward career mobility for the nurses [20–22].

The biggest challenge for CALD nurses in Finland is the recognition of their qualifications obtained abroad. Non-EU nurses, particularly those from the Philippines and other nationalities, experience many obstacles [7]. In particular, the linguistic challenge has been noted as an obstacle to securing an RN position, practising nursing, career development, and work well-being [20–22].

According to Valvira—an institution operating under the Ministry of Social Affairs and Health—acting as the national health supervisory authority of Finland, CALD nurses require the attainment of at least Level 3 according to the Common European Framework of Reference for Languages in terms of the proficiency level of Finnish or Swedish [54]. This, together with complicated re-certification procedures, poses serious barriers to pursuing professional advancement for CALD nursing staff. For example, nurses from EU member states, such as Spain, are afforded a far easier process of recognition under EU Directive 55/2013. CALD nurses often face additional bridging courses.

The bridging education programmes are one of the best available interventions to help alleviate the deskilling phenomenon and incorporate CALD nurses into the workforce [18, 19]. The Finnish government has, in recent years, funded the University of Applied Sciences to offer "top-up" programmes meant to help the credentialing process [54]. These improve professional language proficiency for healthcare purposes, enhance nursing skills, and promote workplace-oriented clinical placements that often provide CALD nurses with future employers [8]. However, the language barrier continues to be a major issue in non-English-speaking countries where English is not the main language, such as Finland and Sweden. Participation in such programmes has the effect of strengthening CALD nurse professional skills and helping socialisation into the new country's healthcare context [18]. The clinical practice component is considered particularly advantageous in providing work experience and building professional relationships. However, many CALD nurses have difficulty finding work as registered nurses [8].

Due to the country's lack of a harmonised nursing curriculum, it is not easy to recognise international competence. There is inequality between the regions, and some of them provide easier ways around CALD nurse integration than others, which gives rise to unequal recognition of foreign qualifications throughout the country [8]. Overcoming such challenges requires changes in recognising foreign qualifications and clearer pathways to be introduced to RN licensure to fully integrate CALD nurses into Finland's nursing human resources [18]. Even though the bridging education programmes provide a very important mechanism for mitigating deskilling, resolving linguistic obstacles and discrepancies in the qualification recognition process requires further action. It is of paramount importance that Finland implements a more work-oriented integration of CALD nurses into her healthcare workforce, contributing to ease the shortage of nursing professionals and developing the professional profile of CALD nurses currently in the country and those recruited in the future [18].

Social and Organisational Integration of CALD Nurses to the Finnish Healthcare Context

Social Integration

Social integration is an important factor determining immigrants' well-being and positive social and economic contribution [4, 10, 14]. However, in many foreign contexts, immigrants have been established to live at the margins of social integration and are exposed to possible social exclusion [14]. Further, negative outcomes that may include isolation and resultant poor mental well-being have been established in instance of low social integration for immigrants [14]. On the contrary, Brissette et al. [4] have demonstrated that positive social integration leads to better health outcomes and resilience even during challenging life events. For instance, a review of studies examining resilience has shown a possible link between support from the host society, social justice, and eventual development of resilience among CALD nurses [10].

The European Union (EU) action plan on integration and inclusion (2021–2027) emphasises the integration and inclusion of immigrants towards the promotion of both strong, cohesive communities and well-being for all. For CALD nurses, same as other immigrants, this means equality in access to opportunities, social and meaningful contribution to society ([11]). For social integration to occur, both the host society and the immigrant have a role to play towards achieving full participation in economic, political, and social contributions [11].

For example, the Finnish Act of the Promotion of Integration (1386/2010) defines integration as an interactive development involving immigrants and the native society and a process that entails social and working life skills (Ministry of Employment and the Economy [36]). Social integration of immigrants in Finland, as stipulated in law, bears both the meaning of integration as the personal development of individual skills and opportunities and the provision of resources that enable an efficient integration process [29]. It is, however, to be noted that traditionally, within the official integration services, much of the efforts have emphasised the integration of refugees, which over time set limitations on the number of immigrants that could access social integration support [29].

However, due to increased migration and the resultant increase in the number of immigrants to Finland in recent years, a need to enhance labour integration and a multisectoral approach to integration has been recognised. Hence, a reform of the Act of the Promotion of Integration (1386/2010) to a more broad-based legal act (681/2023) that comes into force in 2025 has been conducted.

Even though CALD nurses may not be citizens in Finland, their stay is largely long term [30, 56]. Hence, provision for supported social integration is essential for averting negative perceptions and experiences of integration into Finnish society, as established in previous research [41]. Nshom et al. [41] established that immigrants in Finland perceived living and integrating into Finnish society to be challenged by, among others, linguistic challenges, discrimination, racism, and inequality. These factors are further exacerbated by low integration support and a challenge for immigrants accessing what is entitled to their residency status and low expertise to navigate through the interconnected web of integration services [14].

Hence, for a CALD nurse in Finland, the multifaced challenges related to social integration may hinder their smooth and timely integration and expose them to vulnerabilities experienced by immigrants in Finnish society [14, 41]. For instance, the difference in access to employment between natives and immigrants is noticeable and even wider between natives and immigrant female individuals, as well as regional differences, with immigrants in rural areas experiencing poorer integration compared to those in cities [11]. Ndomo [38] further asserts that the Finnish labour market, as currently structured, has created a social understanding that puts immigrant workers, even those highly educated, for instance, CALD nurses, as a subordinate labour force that faces exclusion and unequal integration in the labour market.

In the case of CALD nurse transitioning to the labour market, the Finnish healthcare context may still have much to do in averting the creation of segmentation within its workforce [20–22, 39]. Previous studies on the labour market distribution of CALD nurses have revealed a high presentation within older person care institutions and lower labour mobility to hospital and specialised care [5, 20–22]. Finland has long been able to sustain and replenish its nursing workforce through an intra-country workforce and a small amount of CALD nurses. However, the current global nursing workforce demand and supply trends show that more CALD nurses, even those highly educated, are joining her workforce [20–22, 57]. It is, however, to be noted that both the transition trends to the labour market and integration into the workforce for CALD nurses require special attention [5, 20–22, 57].

Organisational Integration

Global research has established that after CALD nurses transition to working life, they experience a process of organisational integration. This process entails overcoming challenges and attaining organisational citizenship, career development, and retention within a healthcare organisation ([3, 26]; Kamau [18]). Organisational integration of CALD nurses has been defined as a two-way process that entails the nurse and a healthcare organisation [49]. Kamau et al. [20–22] defined CALD nurse organisational integration as a process that involves recognition of competence, structural support, promotion, and acceptance of diversity and overall work well-being.

Further, the process of organisational integration entails the utilisation of integrational strategies and models that support CALD nurse smooth organisational integration [19]. Kamau et al. [19] established that organisational integration strategies and models used towards supporting a CALD nurse can be classified into three: I) intra-organisational strategies and models that are organisational specific and are tailored around a healthcare organisation operation model and culture; II) sociocultural strategies and models used to harness on multiculturalism and cultural diversity within a healthcare organisation nursing workforce and to meet the cultural and linguistic competence needs of the entire workforce and healthcare organisation; and III) professional development as those strategies and models utilised towards supporting CALD nurse ability to practice nursing, competence development, and eventual career development.

Previous research on the organisational integration of nurses in Finland has largely mapped out both challenges experienced by CALD nurses while navigating through the host context and existent opportunities that can be harnessed if CALD nurses were to be efficiently integrated. Kamau et al. [20–22] explored the experiences of CALD nurses integrating into Finland's nursing workforce. Findings established that the nurses underwent negative experiences related to their racial and ethnic backgrounds, linguistic challenges, lowered career mobility, and even mistrust from colleagues. Findings further showed that CALD nurses required healthcare organisations' support towards a safe work environment, orientation to work, managerial support, and professional and career development [20–22]. Cubelo et al. [7] established that for Filipino CALD nurses working in Finland, their experiences of perceived and experienced challenges related to language, navigating the credentialing process, and as undervalued professionals within the workforce created doubt if the CALD nurses wanted to practice nursing in Finland or continue the migration journey to other healthcare contexts, they considered conducive.

On the other hand, Isakov et al. [16] have explored the role of CALD nurse competence in their organisational integration process to health care in Finland. The findings showed that even though general nursing competence did not differ between the immigrant home context and the Finnish context, the nurses experienced challenges with competence recognition and licensure to practice nursing; this further made their organisational integration process more difficult and even tougher where organisational support strategies were minimal or entirely missing.

The experiences of CALD nurses within the Finnish healthcare context and the resultant organisational integration process were examined from the perspective of organisational readiness to hire, support, and integrate a CALD nurse by Tehy—Finland's largest social and healthcare workers' trade union. The survey concluded that the healthcare sector in Finland is not sufficiently prepared to integrate CALD nurses into their workforce. Largely, the structural support strategies built within a healthcare organisation are missing in many organisations and the nurses have reported experiences of racism and discrimination within the workforce.

To better support CALD nurse's organisational integration in Finland, Kamau [18] developed a hypothetical model of organisational integration through data collection and analysis from CALD nurses [20], nurse educators [21], and nurse leaders [22] within the Finnish context. The hypothetical model has proposed 11 concepts that may support a better CALD nurse integration process, namely (1) effective transition to nursing practice, (2) institutional support, (3) leadership involvement, (4) competence recognition and support, (5) understanding of nurses' roles through integration practices, (6) safe working environment, (7) collegiality, (8) relations, (9) cultural diversity in health care, (10) linguistic diversity, and (11) growth within the organisation [18].

The 11 concepts of organisational integration were developed by synthesising stage and interactionist models of organisational integration. The stage model, which includes the anticipatory, encounter, adjustment, and stabilisation phases within a healthcare organisation (Wanberg [58]), provides a framework for understanding the progression of integration from initial expectations to long-term stabilisation. This may mean that first, a CALD nurse joins a healthcare organisation with both professional and personal competences essential for nursing practice and operating within a healthcare context and their effective transition to nursing practice is essential. At this stage, aspects such as a smooth licensure process, recognition of competence, and CALD nurses' personal attributes, such as motivation to work and resilience, are important [18].

Second, when CALD nurses join a healthcare organisation, they experience the reality of being in a foreign care context and organisation. At this stage, their competence may be challenged, and they experience work-related demands; here, competence recognition and support and institutional and leadership support are essential for integrational success. Third, CALD nurses undergo adjustment, which entails their understanding of roles using integrational practices such as mentorship and preceptorship. For a successful adjustment, a safe working environment that is built on strong collegial virtues and relations with colleagues, patients, and families is vital. Fourth, stabilisation is a stage at which the CALD nurse attains organisational citizenship, anticipates future growth within the organisation, and may experience a higher level of remaining within a healthcare organisation. CALD nurse growth within the organisation is also determined by positive linguistic and cultural diversity experiences within a healthcare context [18].

Theoretical Models of Organisational Integration and Examples in the Case of CALD Nurses

The integration into a new organisational context involves an adaptation process where the newcomer must learn the formal and informal rules of organisational life and demonstrate their competence for the role and the tasks they were hired for (Feldman, [13]). These aspects regard every transition across different contexts and professions. The process of work integration has significant effects on turnover intention and intention to leave the profession, especially when considering the first employment [2]. On the other hand, those who have already faced job changes in their professional careers have developed a competence in managing their adjustment and experience lower turnover outcomes and better organisational integration [1, 12, 52].

The main approaches to designing a successful organisational integration sit in four models: The socialisation tactics model (1), proposed by Van Maanen and Schein [55], is based on the passive role of the new hire responding to socialisation strategies implemented by the organisation. These strategies can be individual or institutional and aim to transmit the organisation's behaviours, values, and norms to the new members. When a CALD nurse is hired, the organisation may assign them a mentor to guide them through expected behaviours, communication styles, and procedures. The nurse passively absorbs the organisational norms through formal training and observing experienced staff. These strategies aim to align the new nurse with the hospital's culture and values without altering them. Only when the socialisation process moves forward, the organisation may decide to switch to more flexible and variable socialisation tactics to provide more freedom to the newcomer.

Stage models (2), including those by Feldman [13], Nicholson [40], and Porter, Lawler, and Hackman [47], describe the socialisation process as articulated in different stages. Each stage is specifically described and requires detailed study to be fully understood. The stages typically include an anticipatory phase, an entry phase, and a change-assimilation phase. When a CALD nurse is hired, they may progress through distinct stages of socialisation, beginning with an anticipatory phase where they form expectations about the workplace. In the entry phase, they start adjusting to the hospital environment and its norms. Finally, in the change-assimilation phase, the nurse fully integrates into the organisational culture, adopting its values and practices.

The interactionist models (3) consider an active role for the new hire in the socialisation process, such as sensemaking [27] and interpersonal relationships [50]. The focus is on the proactive behaviour of the person facing the integration path, actively seeking to adapt and integrate into the new environment. When a CALD nurse is hired, they actively engage in the socialisation process by seeking out information and making sense of the hospital's culture. They build interpersonal relationships with colleagues to better understand expectations and norms. Through this proactive behaviour, the nurse adapts and integrates into the new environment and makes sense of the socialisation process within the own personal and professional development.

The last model (4) is based on the socialisation resources theory (SRT) proposed by Saks and Gruman [51]. This approach articulates the socialisation process in stages, each with specific contents. The SRT emphasises the importance of available resources in the organisational context, such as colleague support and feedback availability, for the success of the integration of the new hire. When a CALD nurse is hired, the hospital may provide specific resources like assigning a supportive peer mentor to guide them through clinical procedures and cultural nuances of patient care. Regular feedback from supervisors helps the nurse understand performance expectations and adjust accordingly. Access to language support services or diversity training sessions further facilitates their successful integration into the hospital's team and workflow. Over time, the resources provided by the organisation foster the newcomer's self-confidence and empowerment by supporting an effective person-organisation fit. The table below summarises the four models, and the following sections describe them in more detail (Table 1).

Socialisation Tactics [55]

Van Maanen and Schein [55] proposed a comprehensive model of organisational socialisation, focusing on the tactics organisations use to integrate new members. This model identifies six socialisation tactics, each representing a continuum of possible strategies. These tactics explain how organisations can influence the experiences and behaviours of new employees as they adjust to their roles and integrate into the organisational culture. The six tactics are:

Individual vs. Collective Socialisation

Individual socialisation: The new employee undergoes socialisation on a one-on-one basis, typically through personal experiences or mentorship. This approach allows for a tailored experience, addressing the specific needs and learning pace of the individual.

Collective socialisation: New employees are socialised in groups, experiencing the socialisation process together. This can include orientation programmes, group

Table 1 Summary of theoretical models of organisational integration

Aspect	Socialisation tactics	Stages/ models	Interactionist models	Socialisation resources theory
Role of the new hire	Passive	Passive	Active	Active
Stages/phases	Not staged	Anticipatory, entry, assimilation	Not staged	Demands–resource-based stages
Key actions	Formal induction programmes, observation	Adapting to each stage	Sensemaking, building relationships	Feedback, resource, availability
Organisational resources	Formal training	Mentorship, feedback	Supportive colleagues	Colleague support, feedback

training sessions, or team-building activities. Collective socialisation fosters a sense of belonging and shared understanding among newcomers.

Formal vs. Informal Socialisation

Formal socialisation: The organisation uses structured and preplanned activities to socialise new employees. Examples include formal training programmes, orientation sessions, and workshops. These activities are explicitly designed to teach new hires about the organisational culture, policies, and procedures.

Informal socialisation: Socialisation occurs through unstructured, on-the-job experiences. New employees learn through observation, interactions with colleagues, and daily work activities. Informal socialisation is less controlled by the organisation and can vary widely depending on the individual's experiences and interactions.

These first two tactics (individual-collective and formal-informal) belong to the organisational **context** as they depend on the interaction between the newcomer and the current employees and the activities planned by the organisation to facilitate the newcomer's adjustment.

Sequential vs. Random Socialisation

Sequential socialisation: The socialisation process follows a specific sequence of steps, with clearly defined stages that new employees must go through. Each stage builds on the previous one, providing a clear roadmap for the socialisation process.

Random socialisation: There is no predetermined order or sequence to the socialisation process. New employees may experience different aspects of the organisation in a nonlinear fashion, depending on opportunities and interactions that arise spontaneously.

Fixed vs. Variable Socialisation

Fixed socialisation: The organisation establishes a set timetable for the socialisation process. New employees know exactly how long each stage will take and when they can expect to move on to the next phase.

Variable socialisation: The timing of the socialisation process is flexible and can vary based on the individual's progress, needs, and circumstances. There is no strict timeline, allowing for adaptability to different learning speeds and situations.

These other two tactics (sequential–random and fixed–variable) define the **content** of the organisational socialisation as they identify (or not) specific steps and schedules to guide the organisational socialisation.

Serial vs. Disjunctive Socialisation

Serial socialisation: Experienced members of the organisation (mentors or role models) guide new employees through the socialisation process. This guidance helps newcomers understand expectations and integrate more smoothly into their roles.

Disjunctive socialisation: New employees do not have formal mentors or role models to follow. They must navigate the socialisation process independently, learning through their own experiences and interactions.

Investiture vs. Divestiture Socialisation

Investiture socialisation: The organisation affirms and values the incoming identity, skills, and perspectives of new employees. This approach encourages new hires to retain their individuality and integrate their unique contributions into the organisational culture.

Divestiture socialisation: The organisation seeks to strip away certain personal characteristics of new employees that are deemed incompatible with the organisational culture. The goal is to force newcomers to fit the existing norms and values of the organisation.

These last two tactics (serial-disjunctive and investiture–divestiture) belong to the social aspects of the organisational socialisation process as they define the social interaction practices within the organisation.

Application and Implications

The combination of these dimensions creates a spectrum of socialisation strategies that organisations can adopt based on their culture, goals, and the nature of the roles. By understanding and strategically applying these tactics, organisations can better manage the integration process, ensuring new employees integrate smoothly and effectively into the organisation. The right balance of these tactics can enhance job satisfaction, organisational commitment, and overall performance of new employees.

Example in Practice

An organisation might use a mix of these tactics to achieve optimal socialisation outcomes. For instance, they might begin with collective and formal socialisation through an initial orientation programme, followed by individual and informal socialisation where mentors provide one-on-one guidance. Over time, the organisation could transition from a sequential and fixed structure to a more random and variable approach, allowing for flexibility as new employees settle into their roles. Throughout this process, an investiture approach can ensure that new hires feel valued and encouraged to contribute their unique perspectives.

Stage Models

Stage models of organisational socialisation describe the process of becoming an integrated and effective member of an organisation through a series of distinct phases. These models highlight the progression of new employees as they navigate their entry and adaptation to the organisational environment. The primary stage models include Feldman's model (1977), Nicholson's model (1984), and Porter, Lawler, and Hackman's model (1975).

Feldman's Model (1977)

Feldman's model outlines three primary stages of socialisation:

I—Anticipatory Socialisation

This stage occurs before the individual joins the organisation. It involves the formation of expectations about the job and the organisation based on prior experiences, socialisation agents (e.g. family, friends, and media), and recruitment activities. In the case of newcomer nurses, also undergraduate clinical placements can be considered as a source of anticipatory socialisation: As undergraduate nurses learn clinical competences, they also learn the organisational behaviours within the host healthcare organisation. However, in the case of CALD nurses, this stage might have taken place in a different cultural and organisational context, and this could represent a challenge in CALD nurses' integration.

II—Encounter Stage

This stage begins when the individual joins the organisation. The newcomer experiences the reality of the job and the organisation, which may confirm or disconfirm pre-existing expectations.

III—Change and Acquisition

During this stage, the newcomer begins to adjust and assimilate into the organisation, mastering necessary skills, and adopting the norms and values of the organisation.

Nicholson's Model (1984)

Nicholson's model focuses on four stages of role transition:

I—Preparation

In this stage, the individual prepares psychologically for entry into the new role. This includes mental preparation and gathering information about the new role and organisation.

II—Encounter

The newcomer directly experiences the new work environment, which may involve unexpected challenges and learning opportunities.

III—Adjustment

This stage involves the active adaptation to the new role, including developing new skills, forming relationships, and understanding organisational norms.

IV—Stabilisation

The individual reaches a stage of equilibrium where they have become proficient in their role and feel integrated into the organisational culture.

Porter, Lawler, and Hackman's Model (1975)

This model emphasises three stages in the socialisation process:

I—Entry

The individual enters the organisation and begins to learn about the organisational culture and expectations.

II—Socialisation

The newcomer undergoes a deeper socialisation process, learning the norms, values, and expected behaviours within the organisation.

III—Role Change

The individual adjusts their behaviour and mindset to fit the role and organisational expectations, achieving a level of competence and satisfaction.

Applications and Implications

Understanding and applying stage models in organisational socialisation can help organisations manage the integration process more effectively, ensuring that new employee's transition smoothly through each stage. This can lead to:

Improved job satisfaction: By managing expectations and providing support at each stage, organisations can enhance job satisfaction.

Increased retention: Effective socialisation reduces turnover by helping employees feel integrated and valued.

Enhanced performance: As new employees progress through the stages, they become more competent and aligned with organisational goals.

Example in Practice

Consider a healthcare organisation onboarding a new nurse:

1. Anticipatory Socialisation (Feldman's Model):

Before joining, the nurse gathers information about the hospital's culture, policies, and expectations through recruitment materials and conversations with current staff. Also, clinical placements during undergraduate education are a meaningful source of anticipatory socialisation into the healthcare organisations.

2. Preparation (Nicholson's Model):

The nurse mentally prepares for the new role, setting realistic expectations based on the information gathered.

3. Encounter Stage (Feldman's Model) / Entry (Porter, Lawler, and Hackman's Model):

Upon joining, the nurse attends an orientation programme, meets colleagues, and starts understanding the practical realities of the job.

4. Adjustment (Nicholson's Model) / Socialisation (Porter, Lawler, and Hackman's Model):

The nurse undergoes hands-on training, receives feedback, and starts integrating into the team, learning the hospital's specific procedures and culture.

5. Change and acquisition (Feldman's Model):

The nurse begins to master necessary skills, adapt behaviours to fit organisational norms and feel more confident in the role.

6. Stabilization (Nicholson's Model) / Role Change (Porter, Lawler, and Hackman's Model):

The nurse achieves proficiency, feels a sense of belonging, and consistently performs well, fully integrated into the hospital's culture.

Interactionist Models

Interactionist models of organisational socialisation emphasise the active role of the new employee in interpreting and adapting to their new organisational environment. These models focus on the interactions between the newcomer and their colleagues, as well as the subjective processes of meaning-making and identity formation. Key models include Louis' sensemaking theory (1980) and Reichers' interpersonal relationships model (1987).

Sensemaking Theory [27]

Sensemaking theory suggests that newcomers actively interpret and make sense of their new environment through ongoing interactions and experiences. The process involves:

I—Surprise and Sensemaking

Newcomers may experience surprises or discrepancies between their expectations and the reality of the organisation. This is also known as transition shock (Duchscher and Windey, 20+18).

II—Information Seeking

Newcomers actively seek information to reduce uncertainty and ambiguity.

III—Sensemaking Cycles

Newcomers repeatedly cycle through stages of experiencing surprises, making sense of them, and adjusting their behaviour accordingly.

IV—Identity Construction

Newcomers construct their professional identity through their interpretations and interactions within the organisation.

Interpersonal Relationships Model [50]

Reichers' model emphasises the importance of social relationships in the socialisation process. The key components include:

I—Social Exchange

Newcomers build relationships with colleagues and supervisors, exchanging information, support, and resources.

II—Social Integration

The degree to which newcomers feel accepted and integrated into the organisational social fabric.

III—Interpersonal Influence

The influence that established members have on newcomers through modelling, feedback, and social reinforcement.

IV—Social Support

The emotional, informational, and instrumental support provided by colleagues to help newcomers adjust.

Applications and Implications

Interactionist models highlight the dynamic and reciprocal nature of the integration process, emphasising the role of both the organisation and the newcomer in achieving successful integration. Applications and implications include:

Active engagement: Encouraging newcomers to actively seek information and build relationships can lead to more effective socialisation.

Tailored support: Providing individualised support based on newcomers' needs and interactions can enhance their adjustment and performance.

Enhanced social integration: Fostering a supportive and inclusive organisational culture can facilitate social integration and reduce turnover.

In the case of CALD nurses, the interactionist model interacts with a wider sensemaking process in which the CALD nurses develop a wider process embedded into their personal and professional development, as the organisation integration is often part of a wider societal process of integration.

Example in Practice

1. Surprise and Sensemaking (Louis' Sensemaking Theory):

   The nurse encounters unexpected challenges with the hospital's electronic health record (EHR) system and specific clinical protocols, prompting a sensemaking process to understand the reasons behind these practices.
2. Information Seeking (Louis' Sensemaking Theory):

   The nurse actively seeks information by asking colleagues questions, attending training sessions on the EHR system and clinical protocols, and reviewing hospital documentation to understand the organisation's expectations and processes.
3. Social Exchange (Reichers' Interpersonal Relationships Model):

   The nurse builds relationships with team members through daily interactions, by participating in team meetings, and by engaging in informal discussions during breaks or after shifts.
4. Sensemaking Cycles (Louis' Sensemaking Theory):

   The nurse repeatedly experiences new surprises, reflects on them, and adjusts their behaviour, continuously refining their understanding of the hospital's practices and improving their performance.
5. Social Integration (Reichers' Interpersonal Relationships Model):

   Over time, the nurse feels more accepted and integrated into the healthcare team, contributing to patient care discussions and receiving positive feedback from colleagues and supervisors.
6. Interpersonal Influence and Social Support (Reichers' Interpersonal Relationships Model)

   Experienced nurses serve as role models, providing feedback and support and helping the new nurse navigate complex clinical tasks and build confidence in their role.

Socialisation Resources Theory (SRT) [51]

The socialisation resources theory (SRT) proposed by Saks and Gruman [51] integrates concepts from the job demands–resources (JD-R) model to explain the socialisation process. This theory emphasises the role of resources available to newcomers during socialisation, which can facilitate successful adjustment and integration. The key resources identified are structural, social, and personal.

1. Structural resources: These are the formal mechanisms and supports provided by the organisation to aid in the socialisation process, for example, role clarity, in order to establish clear communication about job expectations, responsibilities, and performance criteria, and organisational support mechanisms such as onboarding programmes, training sessions, and accessible managerial support.
2. Social resources: These include the social interactions and networks that newcomers develop within the organisation. It is important to ensure networking

opportunities for newcomers to build relationships and establish professional networks within the organisation and constructive feedback from peers and supervisors which helps newcomers understand their progress and areas for improvement.

3. Personal resources: These are the individual attributes and skills that newcomers bring to the organisation, which can facilitate their socialisation, for example, self-efficacy as the newcomer's belief in their ability to perform job tasks effectively and the newcomer's ability to adjust to new situations, roles, and environments.

Applications and Implications

The SRT highlights the importance of providing adequate resources to newcomers to ensure successful integration. The applications and implications of this theory include:

Enhanced onboarding programmes: Developing comprehensive onboarding programmes that provide clear role expectations, training, and support.

Mentorship and networking: Facilitating mentorship programmes and opportunities for newcomers to build social networks.

Ongoing feedback and support: Establishing regular feedback mechanisms and ensuring continuous support from supervisors and colleagues.

Fostering personal development: Encouraging self-efficacy and adaptability through challenging tasks, recognition, and supportive transitions.

Example in Practice

Consider a hospital onboarding a new nurse:

1. Role clarity and support (structural resources)

   The hospital provides the nurse with a detailed job description, including specific duties, responsibilities, and performance expectations. The nurse participates in an onboarding programme that includes comprehensive training on hospital protocols, electronic health record systems, and patient care procedures.
2. Networking and feedback (social resources):

   The nurse is paired with an experienced nurse mentor who provides guidance and support. The hospital organises team-building activities and social events to help the RN build relationships with colleagues. Regular feedback sessions are established to discuss the RN's progress, address any challenges, and identify areas for improvement.
3. Self-Efficacy and adaptability (personal resources):

   The nurse is assigned initial tasks that are appropriately challenging to build confidence and demonstrate competence. The hospital recognises the RN's achievements during staff meetings and provides support during transitions to different units or shifts.

By applying the principles of SRT, the hospital ensures that the new nurse receives the necessary structural, social, and personal resources to facilitate a smooth and successful integration into the healthcare setting. This comprehensive approach helps the nurse feel supported, competent, and valued, ultimately enhancing job satisfaction and performance.

Successful Approaches Towards the Support of CALD Nurses Within the Finnish Healthcare Context

Research has developed and tested several successful approaches to support CALD nurses and nursing students in Finnish health care. A key strategy is the implementation of structured mentorship programmes [43, 45], specifically designed to prepare mentors for effectively working with CALD nurses and students in clinical settings. These programmes emphasise the importance of mentors understanding their mentees' cultural backgrounds and beliefs, as this fosters trust and promotes a productive mentoring relationship.

To achieve this, mentors must be aware of their biases and actively address any prejudices, ethnocentric views, or stereotypes they may hold [44]. Respect for the diversity of cultural values is essential, and mentors are encouraged to gather reliable information about a student's cultural background through discussions or portfolios. This approach allows mentors to tailor their support to the individual needs of each student.

Engaging in ongoing learning and demonstrating genuine interest in the mentee's culture strengthen the mentor–student relationship. Communication plays a vital role in this process, requiring understanding verbal and non-verbal cues, which can vary significantly between cultures. For example, in some cultures, maintaining eye contact is seen as respectful, while in others, it may be perceived as confrontational. By fostering open communication and creating an environment where students feel comfortable expressing their needs, mentors can help ensure that cultural differences are acknowledged and understood.

Additionally, mentors are responsible for creating a safe and supportive environment, both physically and emotionally, where students can share concerns and feel valued [31]. Providing constructive feedback and facilitating the integration of students into the nursing team promote a sense of belonging and contribute to a positive and inclusive learning atmosphere that supports students' overall success and well-being [32]. To develop these capabilities, mentors' competence must be enhanced through targeted education, leadership support for ongoing growth, and a work environment that values and fosters a receptive and open atmosphere [48, 53]. The receptive culture of staff towards competence development and growth creates a more inclusive environment by increasing awareness and reducing cultural misunderstandings in healthcare settings [33].

Additionally, language support plays a critical role in the successful integration of CALD nurses in Finland. Mikkonen et al.'s [30] research emphasises the importance of offering comprehensive language training, covering general Finnish language skills and healthcare-specific terminology. This dual-focus approach is essential for building the confidence of CALD nurses, enabling them to communicate effectively and perform proficiently in the workplace. According to the latest research, highly advanced technology solutions developed for CALD nursing students to enhance their language and clinical learning were effective and supportive [34]. The study's key findings revealed that human-centred extended reality (XR) significantly enhanced CALD nursing students' learning in clinical conditions by providing immersive, interactive experiences that improve practical skills, knowledge retention, and confidence in a safe, simulated environment. The study highlights the promise of human-centred XR in healthcare education by offering immersive simulations that allow students to practice clinical skills in a risk-free environment, enhancing both learning outcomes and confidence. This technology holds the potential for creating more accessible and scalable training solutions, enabling personalised, hands-on learning experiences without the constraints of traditional clinical settings.

In addition to language training, fostering collaborative learning environments where CALD nurses work alongside Finnish-educated nurses has proven to be beneficial [23, 28]. These collaborative settings help create a sense of community, where CALD nurses can engage in peer learning and receive support. Peer support networks also provide a platform for CALD nurses to share their experiences and challenges, reducing feelings of isolation and promoting job satisfaction [46]. Tailored orientation programmes specifically designed for CALD nurses are another critical factor in their integration. These programmes address clinical competences and cover the practical aspects of living and working in Finland, including navigating legal requirements and understanding the country's social systems [19]. Such orientation programmes ensure that CALD nurses have the knowledge and skills they need to thrive professionally and personally.

Moreover, professional development opportunities are pivotal in helping CALD nurses advance their careers. Offering pathways for continuous learning allows CALD nurses to align their skills with the demands of the Finnish healthcare system. These opportunities also support CALD nurses in meeting the licensing and regulatory requirements to practice in Finland, ensuring their long-term career growth.

These approaches have proven to be both empirically effective and theoretically consistent with all the organisational socialisation models previously presented. When embedded into the organisational practices, they represent a comprehensive effort to support the integration and professional development of CALD nurses in Finland. Fostering an inclusive work environment that values diversity, these strategies help CALD nurses succeed and contribute meaningfully to the healthcare system.

Conclusion, Future Directions, and Challenges

In conclusion, the integration of culturally and linguistically diverse (CALD) nurses into the Finnish healthcare system is a complex but essential process that requires strategic focus and multifaceted support. With Finland facing a growing shortage of nursing professionals due to an ageing population and workforce constraints, CALD nurses are increasingly seen as a vital resource to ensure safe and quality nursing care. However, for CALD nurses to fully contribute to the system, challenges related to recruitment, credentialing, integration, and reskilling must be addressed. It is crucial that the Finnish healthcare sector develops clear and streamlined pathways of organisational and professional integration for CALD nurses, including recognition of their foreign qualifications and support in overcoming linguistic barriers. Without these efforts, the professional expertise of CALD nurses remains underutilised, which make difficult for CALD nurses and healthcare organisations to work at their full potential, and this could further exacerbate workforce shortages.

Furthermore, organisational integration plays a key role in ensuring CALD nurses can successfully transition into their roles. This process extends beyond formal employment and requires healthcare organisations to foster an inclusive and a supportive environment. Structured mentorship programmes, ongoing professional development opportunities, and comprehensive language training are pivotal for facilitating this transition. Organisational models of integration, which focus on both individual and institutional roles, are critical in helping CALD nurses navigate their new work environments and build meaningful professional relationships. By recognising and valuing the cultural and linguistic diversity of these nurses, healthcare institutions can enhance team cohesion and promote a safe, positive work culture.

Ultimately, the successful integration of CALD nurses is beneficial not only for the nurses themselves but also for the sustainability and quality of health care in Finland. Addressing the systemic barriers to their integration will help ensure that CALD nurses can contribute their full potential to the healthcare system. In turn, this will improve patient care outcomes and help mitigate the ongoing nursing shortage. Investing in these integration strategies is a long-term solution that strengthens the healthcare workforce while also promoting diversity and inclusion in Finnish society.

References

1. Bauer TN, Morrison EW, Callister RR. Organizational socialization: a review and directions for future research. Res Pers Hum Resour Manag. 1998;16:149–214.
2. Bauer TN, Bodner T, Erdogan B, Truxillo DM, Tucker JS. Newcomer adjustment during organizational socialization: a meta-analytic review of antecedents, outcomes, and methods. J Appl Psychol. 2007;92(3):707–21. https://doi.org/10.1037/0021-9010.92.3.707.
3. Berry JW, Phinney JS, Sam DL, Vedder P. Immigrant youth: acculturation, identity, and adaptation. Appl Psychol. 2006;55(3):303–32.
4. Brissette I, Cohen S, Seeman TE. Measuring social integration and social networks. In: Cohen S, Underwood L, Gottlieb B, editors. Social support measurement and intervention. New York: Oxford University Press; 2000. p. 53–85.
5. Calenda D, Pitkänen P, Sippola A. Integration of foreign-born nurses in finnish social and health care organizations: evidences, challenges and responses. J Immigr Refug Stud. 2018;17(2):152–67. https://doi.org/10.1080/15562948.2018.1428843.

6. Cubelo F. Internationally educated nurses' role in climate change: sustainability and mitigation practices. Public Health Nurs (Boston, Mass). 2023;40(4):585–9. https://doi.org/10.1111/phn.13185.
7. Cubelo F, Langari MNM, Jokiniemi K, Turunen H. Recognition of nursing qualification and credentialing pathway of Filipino nurses in Finland: a qualitative study. Int Nurs Rev. 2023;71(3):661.
8. Cubelo F, Parviainen A, Kohanová D. The impact of bridging education programs on internationally educated nurses becoming registered nurses in high-income countries: a mixed-methods systematic review. Int Nurs Rev. 2024;72(2):e13038. https://doi.org/10.1111/inr.13038.
9. Cubelo F. Policy reform on the qualification pathway of internationally educated nurses in greenland and its relationship with the danish system: a qualitative discourse analysis. Policy, Politics, & Nursing Practice. 2024;25(3):172–181. https://doi.org/10.1177/15271544241245975.
10. Dahl K, Nortvedt L, Schrøder J, Bjørnnes AK. Internationally educated nurses and resilience: a systematic literature review. Int Nurs Rev. 2022;69(3):405–15.
11. European Commission. Action plan on Integration and Inclusion 2021–2027. In: Communication from the Commission to the European Parliament, the Council, the European Economic and Social Committee and the Committee of the Regions; 2020. p. 758.
12. Feldman DC. A contingency theory of socialization. Adm Sci Q. 1976;21(3):433–52. https://doi.org/10.2307/2391853.
13. Feldman DC. A contingency theory of socialization. Adm Sci Q. 1977;21(3):433–52. https://doi.org/10.2307/2391853.
14. Grigaityte I. Social integration, psychological well-being, and proactive attitudes towards the integration of immigrants in a sample of the Swedish-speaking population in Western Finland. Åbo Akademi University; 2022. https://urn.fi/URN:ISBN:978-952-12-4169-7
15. ICN. Investing in the nursing workforce for health system effectiveness. 2021. https://www.icn.ch/sites/default/files/2023-07/ICN_Recover-to-Rebuild_report_EN.pdf.
16. Isakov T, Kamau S, Koskenranta M, Kuivila H, Oikarainen A, Ropponen P, Mikkonen K. Culturally and linguistically diverse nurses' experiences of how competence facilitates integration into the working environment: a qualitative study. Nurse Educ Pract. 2023;67(103):553.
17. Jester R. Editorial – Global shortage of nurses – Rebecca Jester for May 2023 issue. Int J Orthop Trauma Nurs. 2023;49(101):018. https://doi.org/10.1016/j.ijotn.2023.101018.
18. Kamau S. Organisational integration of culturally and linguistically diverse nurses:a hypothetical model. 2024. https://oulurepo.oulu.fi/bitstream/handle/10024/49105/nbnfioulu-202404102635.pdf?sequence=1&isAllowed=y.
19. Kamau S, Koskenranta M, Kuivila H, Oikarainen A, Tomietto M, Juntunen J, Mikkonen K. Integration strategies and models to support transition and adaptation of culturally and linguistically diverse nursing staff into healthcare environments: an umbrella review. Int J Nurs Stud. 2022;136(104):377.
20. Kamau S, Koskenranta M, Isakov TM, Kuivila H, Oikarainen A, Tomietto M, Mikkonen K. Culturally and linguistically diverse registered nurses' experiences of integration into nursing workforce–a qualitative descriptive study. Nurse Educ Today. 2023a;121(105):700. https://doi.org/10.1016/j.nedt.2022.105700.
21. Kamau S, Oikarainen A, Kiviniitty N, Koskenranta M, Kuivila H, Tomietto M, Mikkonen K. Nurse leaders' experiences of how culturally and linguistically diverse registered nurses integrate into healthcare settings: an interview study. Int J Nurs Stud. 2023b;146(104):559.
22. Kamau S, Oikarainen A, Juntunen MM, Koskenranta M, Kuivila H, Tomietto M, Mikkonen K. Nurse educators' views of integrating culturally and linguistically diverse future registered nurses into healthcare settings: a qualitative descriptive study. J Adv Nurs. 2023c;79(9):3412–25.
23. Kemppainen E, Kuha S, Koskenranta M, Mikkonen K, Kanste O. Nursing line-managers' experiences of emotional intelligence management in multicultural work communities in the social and health care sector (in Finnish). Nurs Sci. 2024.
24. Kesti R, Kanste O, Konttila J, Oikarinen A. Quality of working life of employees in public healthcare organization in Finland: a cross-sectional study. Nurs Open. 2023;10(9):6455–64. https://doi.org/10.1002/nop2.1896.

25. Klemetti R, Vuorenmaa M, Heino A, Raussi-Lehto E, Kalliolehto J, Kaarakainen M, Gissler M. Integration of maternity care as a part of social welfare and health care reform in Finland. Int J Integr Care. 2023;23(S1):556. https://doi.org/10.5334/ijic.ICIC23204.
26. Lai DW, Shankar J, Khalema E. Unspoken skills and tactics: essentials for immigrant professionals in integration to workplace culture. J Int Migr Integr. 2017;18(3):937–59.
27. Louis MR. Surprise and sense making: what newcomers experience in entering unfamiliar organisational settings. Adm Sci Q. 1980;25(2):226–51.
28. Luukkonen AL, Kuivila H, Kaarlela V, Koskenranta M, Kaučič BM, Riklikiene O, Vizcaya-Moreno F, Pérez-Cañaveras RM, Filej B, Oikarainen A, Kääriäinen M, Mikkonen K. Mentors' cultural competence at mentoring culturally and linguistically diverse nursing students in clinical practice: an international cross-sectional study. Nurse Educ Pract. 2023;70(103):658. https://doi.org/10.1016/j.nepr.2023.103658.
29. Martikainen T, Valtonen K, Wahlbeck Ö. The social integration of immigrants in Finland. In: International perspectives: integration and inclusion; 2012. p. 127–46.
30. Mikkonen K, Elo S, Kuivila HM, Tuomikoski AM, Kääriäinen M. Culturally and linguistically diverse healthcare students' experiences of learning in a clinical environment: a systematic review of qualitative studies. Int J Nurs Stud. 2016;54:173–87.
31. Mikkonen K, Elo S, Tuomikoski A, Kaariainen M. Mentor experiences of international healthcare students' learning in a clinical environment: a systematic review. Nurse Educ Today. 2016a;40:87–94. https://doi.org/10.1016/j.nedt.2016.02.013.
32. Mikkonen K, Elo S, Miettunen J, Saarikoski M, Kaariainen M. Clinical learning environment and supervision of international nursing students: a cross-sectional study. Nurse Educ Today. 2017;52:73–80. https://doi.org/10.1016/j.nedt.2017.02.017.
33. Mikkonen K, Merilainen M, Tomietto M. Empirical model of clinical learning environment and mentoring of culturally and linguistically diverse nursing students. J Clin Nurs. 2020;29(3–4):653–61. https://doi.org/10.1111/jocn.15112.
34. Mikkonen K, Ferdinando H, Sobocinski M, Kuivila H, Pramila-Savukoski S, Vhitehead T, Ropponen P, Myllylä T, Paunonen J, Halili E, Koutonen J, Taikina-Aho JM, Siipo A, Järvelä A. How does human-centred extended reality support healthcare students' learning in clinical conditions? In: Säreströniemi M, et al., editors. Digital health and wireless solutions, NCDHWS 2024. Communications in computer and information science, vol. 2083. Cham: Springer; 2024. https://doi.org/10.1007/978-3-031-59080-1_13.
35. Ministry of Economic Affairs and Employment. New studies provide data on promotion of international recruitment in health and social services sector. 2023. https://valtioneuvosto.fi/en/-//1410877/new-studies-provide-data-on-promotion-of-international-recruitment-in-health-and-social-services-sector.
36. Ministry of Employment and the Economy. 2010. https://www.finlex.fi/en/laki/kaannokset/2010/en20101386.pdf.
37. Ministry of Social Affairs and Health. Government proposal for health and social services reform and related legislation adopted by Parliament. 2021. https://valtioneuvosto.fi/en/-/1271139/government-proposal-for-health-and-social-services-reform-and-related-legislation-adopted-by-parliament.
38. Ndomo Q. The working underclass: Highly educated migrants on the fringes of the Finnish labour market. University of Jyväskylä; 2024.
39. Ndomo Q, Bontenbal I, Lillie NA. Essential? COVID-19 and highly educated Africans in Finland's segmented labour market. Int J Sociol Soc Policy. 2023;43(3/4):339–55. https://doi.org/10.1108/IJSSP-06-2022-0171.
40. Nicholson N. A theory of work role transitions. Adm Sci Q. 1984;29(2):172–91.
41. Nshom E, Sadaf S, Khalimzoda I. Perceived challenges living and integrating into Finnish society: a study among immigrants in Finland. J Intercult Commun. 2022;22(3):31–42. https://doi.org/10.36923/jicc.v22i3.82.
42. OECD.(2023). State of Health in the EU, Finland Country Health Profile 2023. https://health.ec.europa.eu/document/download/69be51c9-628e-467e-9825-50eb23559f17_en?filename=2023_chp_fi_english.pdf.

43. Oikarainen A, Mikkonen K. Competence in mentoring culturally and linguistically diverse nursing students. In: Mikkonen K, Riklikiene O, Filej B, Kaucic M, editors. Advanced mentorship competences, Modules I-III of advanced mentorship competences. E-publication. Visoka zdravstven sola; 2021. ISBN 978-961-92865-9-3.
44. Oikarainen A, Mikkonen K, Tuomikoski A, Elo S, Pitkanen S, Ruotsalainen H, Kaariainen M. Mentors' competence in mentoring culturally and linguistically diverse nursing students during clinical placement. J Adv Nurs. 2018;74(1):148–59. https://doi.org/10.1111/jan.13388.
45. Oikarainen A, Kaarlela V, Heiskanen M, Taam-Ukkonen M, Lehtimaja I, Kärsämänoja T, Tuomikoski AM, Kääriäinen M, Tomietto M, Mikkonen M. Educational intervention to support development of mentors' competence in mentoring culturally and linguistically diverse nursing students: a quasi-experimental study. Nurse Educ Today. 2022;116:105424. https://doi.org/10.1016/j.nedt.2022.105424.
46. Paatela S, Pohjamies N, Kanste O, Haapa T, Oikarainen A, Kääriäinen M, Mikkonen K. Registered nurses' cultural orientation competence for culturally and linguistically diverse nurses in the hospital setting: a cross-sectional study. J Adv Nurs. 2024;80(2):707–20. https://doi.org/10.1111/jan.15829.
47. Porter LW, Lawler EE, Hackman JR. Behavior in Organisations. McGraw-Hill; 1975.
48. Pramila-Savukoski S, Juntunen J, Tuomikoski A, Kaariainen M, Tomietto M, Kaucic BM, et al. Mentors' self-assessed competence in mentoring nursing students in clinical practice: a systematic review of quantitative studies. J Clin Nurs. 2020;29(5–6):684–705. https://doi.org/10.1111/jocn.15127.
49. Ramji Z, Etowa J. Workplace integration: key considerations for internationally educated nurses and employers. Adm Sci. 2018;8(1):2.
50. Reichers AE. An interactionist perspective on newcomer socialisation rates. Acad Manag Rev. 1987;12(2):278–87.
51. Saks AM, Gruman JA. Getting newcomers engaged: the role of socialisation tactics. J Manag Psychol. 2012;27(3):383–402.
52. Taylor JC, Westcott M, Bartlett JL. The impact of socialization tactics on newcomer adjustment in healthcare settings. J Nurs Adm. 2001;31(7–8):393–404. https://doi.org/10.1097/00005110-200107000-00010.
53. Tuomikoski A, Ruotsalainen H, Mikkonen K, Kaariainen M. Nurses' experiences of their competence at mentoring nursing students during clinical practice: a systematic review of qualitative studies. Nurse Educ Today. 2020;85(104):258. https://doi.org/10.1016/j.nedt.2019.104258.
54. Valvira. Demonstrating sufficient language proficiency. Valvira; n.d.. Retrieved September 30, 2024, from https://valvira.fi/en/rights-to-practise/sufficient-language-proficiency.
55. Van Maanen J, Schein EH. Toward a theory of organisational socialisation. In: Staw BM, editor. Research in organisational behavior, vol. 1. JAI Press; 1979. p. 209–64.
56. Vartiainen P, Pitkänen P, Asis M, Raunio P, Koskela M. International recruitment of Filipino nurses to Finland – expectations and realities. J Popul Soc Stud. 2016;24(1):30–46.
57. Wesołowska K, Hietapakka L, Elovainio M, Aalto A, Kaihlanen A, Heponiemi T. The association between cross-cultural competence and well-being among registered native and foreign-born nurses in Finland. PLoS One. 2018;13(12):e0208761. https://doi.org/10.1371/journal.pone.0208761.
58. Wanberg, Connie R (ed.). The oxford handbook of organizational socialization, oxford library of psychology. 2012. https://doi.org/10.1093/oxfordhb/9780199763672.001.0001.

More than 90 years of Nursing Migration to the United Kingdom: Have We Really Learnt Anything?

John Unsworth and Alwin Puthenpurakal

Global Shortage

Internationally educated nurses (IENs) now make up just under a quarter of all registered nurses in the United Kingdom (UK). In 2024, more than 200,000 IENs were on the Nursing and Midwifery Council (NMC) register representing 23.8% of the total registrants [1]. The rate of international recruitment is slowing predominantly because of cost-saving measures in the health service rather than because the vacancies are now all filled [2]. The largest group of IENs are from India (more than 67,576) followed by the Philippines (50,180) with the remainder having been recruited from various countries including some 'red list' countries [3] including Nigeria and Ghana [4].

At this point, it is worth outlining that the United Kingdom of Great Britain and Northern Ireland is made up of four countries: England, Wales, Scotland and Northern Ireland. Since the late 1990s, each of the countries has had its own government that controls certain devolved matters including health. In 1922, Ireland became independent save for six counties in the North which were partitioned and remained part of the United Kingdom.

J. Unsworth (✉)
Northumbria University, Newcastle-upon-Tyne, UK
e-mail: john.unsworth@northumbria.ac.uk

A. Puthenpurakal
University of Greenwich, London, UK
e-mail: A.Puthenpurakal@greenwich.ac.uk

R. El Moubadder et al. (eds.), *Globalization and Integration of Internationally Educated Nurses: A Comprehensive Analysis*,
https://doi.org/10.1007/978-3-032-01106-0_4

Impact

In terms of workforce shortages, analysis of the latest data shows that the National Health Service (NHS) in England is short of just under 28,000 registered nurses and midwives [5]. As highlighted earlier, this vacancy rate persists despite international recruitment for more than two decades and exists even though further international recruitment has been paused. Across the United Kingdom, there are varying degrees of nursing vacancies. In Scotland, the current data shows more than 2000 whole-time equivalent vacancies despite recruitment and a shift towards a greater number of support worker roles [6]. While in Wales, there are 1778 vacancies across nursing and midwifery [7]. Finally, in Northern Ireland 1852 vacancies exist at the time of writing [8].

Reasons for the Domestic Shortage of Nurses

Workforce planning across the UK health services has been a bit of a hit-and-miss affair leading to both under- and oversupply at various points since the inception of the National Health Service in 1948. Birch [9] argues that part of the problem with workforce projections is that they assume that demand will remain fairly static except for demographic changes in the population. We now know of course that demand is never static and that a failure or issue in any part of the system can increase demand in another part. For example, in England alone primary care and community services see more than 1.4 million people per day [10] but their own workforce issues and underinvestment have resulted in pressures where people fail to get an appointment. A proportion of these people will attend the emergency department to be seen with unanticipated increased demand on those services.

However, anticipating the demand for care is only one part of the workforce planning conundrum; planners also need to consider how services will be delivered in the future and the type of practitioner they think will be needed to work in such services [11]. This also represents another challenge as often policy objectives such as moving care from hospital to community services is not achieved and therefore the workforce plan to have more community-based practitioners is left with an over-supply problem [12].

The reasons for the current domestic shortage of nurses can be broadly grouped into three categories. These are a failure to attract and educate enough nurses (a supply failure), a failure to retain the existing workforce (a retention failure) and the age of the existing workforce resulting in loss because of retirement (a succession failure). We will briefly examine each of these in turn.

Failure to Ensure Workforce Supply

The failure to ensure workforce supply is complex as it is not purely about workforce forecasting. Palmer [13] describes how if the issue was purely down to forecasting, then it would be wrong in both directions with oversupply at some points and undersupply at others. This is certainly true of NHS workforce planning in the 1980s [14] but since then we have seen consistent undersupply. In the United Kingdom, the cost of training a nurse is around £60,000 [15], and while some of this cost falls to the individual who repays a student loan, the NHS bears the cost for placement provision, travel and some financial support for the individual. As a result, the Treasury is cautious about growing student numbers because of the potential increased cost which could be coupled with adverse media coverage when nurses fail to secure employment at the end of the course. There are also concerns about value for money with attrition from nursing courses being as high as 25% [16] and the percentage of newly qualified nurses leaving within 5 years of registration has risen by 67% [17]. This caution was cast aside when the Conservative government developed the NHS Long Term Workforce Plan (LTWP) in 2023 [18]. The LTWP projected that in England training places for adult nurses alone would grow by 92% taking the total to almost 38,000 by 2031/32. However, the plan was unfunded and is now under review by the Labour government who have inherited a range of unfunded commitments alongside a sluggish economy. It is also seen as unsuitable for the NHS transformation envisaged by the new government [19]. The plan was also hit by a reduction in applications for nursing programmes which meant the baseline was not met [20]. This reduction followed a growth in applications during the pandemic [21] and is thought to be associated with adverse publicity about low pay and industrial action [22].

While the proportion of 18-year-olds entering nursing has increased in recent years (e.g. up from 19.1% in 2016 to 22.2% in 2017), new entrants are predominantly from other age groups [23]. The average age of a student studying nursing is 29 years, and a third of those enrolled on a nursing degree are over 35 years [24]. This reflects the fact that nursing has focused on widening participation to more mature students and those with experience although work in this area still has some way to go before it is truly representative of the population the health service serves [25].

Several authors [26, 27] cite the Conservative government's decision to end the training bursary in England in 2017 as one of the main policy decisions which impacted on workforce supply. While it is true that in the year following withdrawal recruitment to nursing courses suffered with a 23% reduction in 2017 [28], the numbers recovered and grew from 2020 onwards [29]. This is only part of the picture as applications from more mature students (defined as 21 and older) continued to decline [29] and various measures were introduced to address the withdrawal of the bursary including a cost-of-living grant in 2020 [30]. However, Gershlick and Charlesworth [31] describe how despite the move to student loans, which need to be repaid over a 30–40-year period by the individual once working, student numbers on nursing programmes grew between 2019 and 2022.

Failure to Retain the Existing Workforce

The Nursing and Midwifery Council [32] reported that while a record number of nurses joined the register in 2022, a total of 27,000 nurses also left the register many earlier than planned because of burnout, exhaustion, a lack of support from colleagues, staffing levels and concerns about the quality of care. Of significant concern was that 85% of leavers said that they were unlikely to ever return in the future. The NMC [32] reports that out of the record 52,148 new registrants in 2022/23, around half were internationally educated nurses (25,006). While the increased numbers of new nurses were welcomed, the fact that 27,000 left the register in the same period meant that the numbers were having a reduced impact in addressing the shortage of qualified nurses.

Two groups of staff are of major concern in terms of retention [33]. The first group are those early-career nurses who are in the first few years of their career who tend to leave after 5 years of service [34] and late-career or more experienced nurses who are approaching retirement age [35]. Both groups of nurses are essential to the delivery of safe and effective care. Early-career nurses are essential to address the increasing age of the NHS workforce in the United Kingdom [33], while more experienced (late-career) nurses are important because of their rich skills and experience and their ability to mentor and nurture new recruits. A workforce which is built around early-career nurses and internationally educated nurses is likely to represent a considerable risk to patient safety because of what is known as the 'rookie factor' [36].

Globally, the COVID-19 pandemic heightened awareness of the global workforce crisis and the threat this posed to population health and health systems. Most major health systems went into the pandemic with a workforce shortfall. Exposure to moral insult and injury, stress, burnout and fatigue during and after the pandemic has undoubtedly exacerbated workforce shortages [37]. However, numerous factors play a part in the retention of the existing workforce. Amongst early-career nurses job satisfaction plays a significant role as does a positive working environment [38]. Interventions which are designed to support the transition into a new role and a career framework alongside preceptorship and mentoring all play a part in retaining nurses [39]. Amongst late-career nurses, flexible working, remuneration and opportunities for continuous professional development are key to staff retention [40].

Size and Shape of the Workforce

The UK National Health Service is the fifth largest employer in the world with more than 1.5 million employees [41]. The NHS workforce is predominantly female (77% of the workforce) although there is a significant gender disparity in role distribution with only 37% of senior NHS roles being occupied by women [42]. The workforce is ethnically and culturally diverse with 26.4% of the workforce being from global majority backgrounds; this rises to around 52% in some regions such as London. Global majority staff are concentrated in lower paid roles with only 11.2% of very senior managers being from the global majority [43].

Kline and Warmington [44] in their report *Too Hot to Handle?* found that the health service was still falling short in terms of tackling race discrimination. The report brought together findings from significant tribunal cases and survey responses from 1327 NHS staff. The survey found that UK-trained staff were more likely than their internationally educated counterparts to raise concerns about discrimination. The most common reason for not raising concerns was a belief that nothing would change (75.7%) and of those who had raised concerns, only 5.4% said that they were taken seriously and the issue was dealt with satisfactorily. Shockingly, the most common outcome to a race discrimination concern was that nothing happened

(42.7%) and that in one in five cases the claim was treated the same way as any other dispute between parties and referred to mediation. In 5% of cases, the individuals who raised the concerns were themselves disciplined. Clearly, NHS organisations have a long way to go to address systemic racism and move beyond denial and obfuscation to fundamentally rooting out racism and racist beliefs.

Given that more than a quarter of the NHS workforce is now from the global majority, the issue of racism and lack of opportunity is a significant stain on the UK health service. The issue of racism runs much deeper than just in the NHS of course and as we will cover in the next section it plays out in immigration policy and how people are treated once they migrate to the United Kingdom.

Immigration

History of Nursing Immigration and Migration

The history of nursing migration is often associated with acute shortages of nurses in the 1940s post-war period but the history of nurses supporting healthcare in the United Kingdom and across the then British Empire goes much further back in history. Rafferty and Solano [45] describe how the Colonial Nursing Association (renamed the Overseas Nursing Association in 1919) recruited more than 8000 nurses to work through the British Empire. The Colonial Nursing Association was formed in 1896 to provide 'white women' to work as nurses in overseas territories. The model was focused on spreading the new approach to nursing education developed by Florence Nightingale [45]. While the Colonial Nursing Association was initially focused on providing nurses to the Empire during the war years, the Colonial Nursing Service moved to recruiting nurses to the United Kingdom [46]. Many nurses moved prior to the 1930s from Ireland to the United Kingdom [47] because of the higher status of nursing and increased opportunities. Migration of nurses from Ireland continued throughout the period from 1920s through to the 1970s. Ryan [48] describes how despite being predominantly white and European, Irish nurses struggled to fully integrate into Britain because of their Irish and predominantly catholic backgrounds.

In the 1930s nurses were among more than 50,000 refugees from Europe who came to Britain to escape fascism and Nazi oppression [49]. The refugees came from Germany, Austria and Czechoslovakia with a smaller number coming from other European countries such as Poland, Norway and Italy. On arrival in the United Kingdom, these nurses faced public opposition and somewhat grudging acceptance [49] because of public concern about the home labour market in a time of high unemployment. In the 1930s many British hospitals faced a shortage of nurses but despite such shortages the government put in place complex regulations determining where and how refugees might be employed [50]. Many of these nurses did not have their qualifications recognised and instead ended up taking employment as nursing assistants. In fact, only 215 nurses of all nationalities were allowed to take up hospital work as probationers or postgraduate nurses between 1935 and 1937 [51].

The pre-World War II experiences of nurses who immigrated to the United Kingdom suggest that there was public concern about them taking jobs from British people despite a continued failure to fill such jobs. In addition, there was also fear of foreigners and indeed in the 1930 antisemitic discrimination. As Gertrude Roberts in an oral history interview with Jane Brooks [51]; p. 79 put it *'there was also a degree of anti-German and antisemitic attitudes: some refugee nurses were clear that they were not accepted at certain famous hospitals because they were "refugees" and "foreign"'*.

Following the creation of the National Health Service in 1948 an acute shortage of doctors and nurses led to further mass overseas recruitment, this time from India and from the West Indies. From 1949 onwards the Ministries of Health and Labour in conjunction with the Colonial Office, the Royal College of Nursing and the General Nursing Council launched campaigns to recruit nursing staff from the Caribbean [52]. Advertisements were placed in local Caribbean newspapers offering up to 3-year contracts for nurses and auxiliary staff. Many of the early recruits joined the UK NHS as part of a Windrush Generation because of the association with one of the first ships to carry immigrants, the Empire Windrush.

By 1955, there was recruitment from more than 16 British colonies and former colonies. Recruitment continued through the 1960s and 1970s with potential recruits for nurse education programmes also being offered opportunities [52]. At the time a two-tier system of nursing registration existed in the United Kingdom with a 3-year State Registered Nurse (SRN) and a shorter practically focused programme for State Enrolled Nurse (SEN). Most Caribbean and Black nurses were placed on the 2-year SEN course despite having the entry qualifications for SRN representing further evidence of racial discrimination [52]. The huge contribution that these nurses made to the successful establishment of the UK NHS has recently been acknowledged [53]. At the same time, it is accepted that the migration to the United Kingdom came at a huge cost to the nurses themselves as they faced both institutional discrimination as well as racism and feeling like a cultural outsider in Britain [54]. The racial discrimination ran deep including preventing nurses from accessing promotion to only applying to the hospital where they were placed in the health system. Olwig [55] describes how immigrants, especially women, were often given denigrated dirty care work. This was true of nurse immigrants who were placed on elderly care wards in patient-facing roles rather than in other areas of nursing practice.

Yeo [56] describes how the nurses from the Caribbean were British subjects with British passports who felt they were coming home to the United Kingdom to support the NHS in its hour of need. This sentiment and the undoubted dreams of those Windrush nurses is accurately reflected in the poem *You called...and we came* [57] which later adorned the National Windrush Monument in London. However, things were to take a darker turn in 2018 in one of the worst political scandals to affect the United Kingdom in a generation [58]. The Windrush Scandal relates to the mistreatment of Caribbean immigrants and their descendants who came to the United Kingdom between 1948 and 1973. Despite the fact they had the right to live and work in the United Kingdom and in fact their descendants were born here, many were detained, denied rights including NHS services and some were even deported because they did not have the necessary documentation [59]. A redress scheme was established but at the time of writing those affected have still not all received compensation.

The United Kingdom has become increasingly multicultural since the 1950s following successive waves of immigration [60]. In 1942, fewer than 5% of the population had actually met someone from an ethnic minority background but by 2021 more than a third of the entire population of England were either migrants themselves or had parents or grandparents from outside of the United Kingdom [61]. As a multicultural nation the nature of society has changed with increasing diversity in terms of music, art, food and religion [62]. Despite progress in the last 20 years, direct or indirect racial discrimination remains widespread with insults, racist jokes, stereotyping and being treated differently affecting 38–47% of individuals from ethnic minority groups [60]. Within the NHS the Workforce Race Equality Standard (WRES) was introduced in 2015 to ensure that staff from Black and minority ethnic backgrounds have access to career opportunities and receive fair treatment in the workplace [63]. The WRES standards have had some success since 2015 with greater representation and an increase in Black and minority ethnic staff in senior NHS roles [64]. However, staff continue to experience racism and indeed in 2023 Michelle Cox won a landmark tribunal for racial discrimination against NHS England [65].

Although significantly smaller in number a few UK-trained nurses leave to work elsewhere in the world. Over time, the range of countries UK nurses emigrate to has changed, and the current countries of choice include the United States, New Zealand and Australia [66]. More common is the loss of internationally educated nurses who have joined the UK register, then deciding to leave for a different country because of better pay and conditions [67].

Policy

Since leaving the European Union, UK immigration policy has undergone significant changes, including the introduction of a points-based system prioritising skilled workers [68, 69]. In 2024, net migration was 728,000 people [70]. Public debate often conflates skilled migration with irregular migration, including asylum seekers fleeing conflict [71]. In 2024, 38,784 irregular arrivals were detected, primarily crossing the English Channel in small boats [72]. Immigration discourse has become increasingly toxic due to confusion between economic migrants, refugees and asylum seekers, despite the United Kingdom's reliance on migration to fill skills gaps and sustain university funding [73]. Since 2012, policies have fostered a 'hostile environment' restricting access to housing, healthcare and employment to deter illegal immigration, though legal migrants are often inadvertently affected [74, 75].

Mobilisation

Internationally educated nurses (IENs) seeking to work in the United Kingdom apply under the Skilled Worker visa, commonly called the Health and Care Worker visa, which exempts them from the Immigration Health Surcharge [68]. The visa application process involves passing an English proficiency test, submitting qualifications to the Nursing and Midwifery Council and completing the computer-based test (CBT) before receiving a Certificate of Sponsorship (CoS) from their employer [76]. The visa application can be submitted 3 months before the job start date, with decisions usually made within 3 weeks.

Upon arrival, nurses typically work as healthcare assistants while completing their registration, which must be finalised within 8 months [77]. They have 12 weeks to take the first attempt at the Objective Structured Clinical Examination (OSCE) and up to three attempts to pass all ten OSCE stations. The OSCE is a high-stakes assessment that contributes to anxiety, and failure results in the withdrawal of the job offer, leading to visa cancellation and a forced return to their home country.

Once registration is achieved, the nurse can work in any of the UK countries and can switch an employer by requesting another Certificate of Sponsorship (CoS) and updating the UK visa agency.

In 2021, the majority of internationally educated nurses arriving in England were from the Philippines (28,521) and India (19,912), followed by European and red list countries like Nigeria (3725), Zimbabwe (2413) and Ghana (1575) [78]. While the NHS Code of Practice prohibits targeted recruitment from red list countries due to their low nurse-to-population ratios, individual nurses can still apply independently [79, 80]. Africa's healthcare worker density (1.55 per 1000) is well below the WHO's recommended threshold (4.45) for Universal Health Coverage, and shortages are expected to worsen, with a projected shortfall of 6.1 million by 2030 [81].

Ethical concerns arise when recruiting from nations experiencing their own nurse shortages. The WHO Global Code of Practice advises against actively recruiting from fragile health systems, leading the United Kingdom to maintain a red list of over 50 countries, including Nigeria and Ghana [79, 82]. UK employers and agencies are prohibited from targeted recruitment in these nations unless a formal government-to-government agreement exists (as seen with Nepal). However, adherence to these guidelines remains complex.

Despite ethical policies, nurses from red list countries increasingly join the NHS, often facilitated by third-party agencies. Nigeria and Ghana were the third and fourth largest contributors of new UK nurse registrants in 2021–2022, with a 25% increase from Nigeria and a 62% rise from Ghana [83]. By mid-2023, international recruitment reached record levels, with nearly as many overseas-trained nurses joining the Nursing and Midwifery Council (NMC) register (15,036) as UK-trained nurses (15,067) [84]. A significant portion of these recruits came from red list countries, raising concerns among NHS leaders and unions about the impact on global healthcare equity.

Palmer at al [78]. estimate that internationally educated nurses stay on average around 12 years; this compares favourably with UK-educated nurses who tend to leave the NHS after 10 years and European Union (EU) nationals who stay around 6 years before departure. It costs between £10,000 and £12,000 to recruit a nurse who is internationally educated which equates to around £1500 a year in terms of the average length of service [78]. Internationally educated nurses therefore represent a good return on investment given that the cost of educating a UK nurse is more than £60,000. In addition, organisations need to factor in agency costs and the risks associated with low registered nurses in terms of patient mortality and complications.

Migration

The term 'hostile environment' refers to a set of stringent UK immigration policies over the past decade aimed at deterring undocumented migrants; these are measures which have also created a climate of fear and bureaucracy affecting many lawful migrant workers [85]. Internationally educated nurses (IENs) in the United Kingdom often feel the spillover effects of this climate. Research by the Institute for Public Policy Research (IPPR) think tank [85] found that the hostile environment has '*helped to foster racism and discrimination*' and even '*erroneously affected people with the legal right to live and work in the UK*'. In practical terms, this means IENs may face difficulties renting housing or accessing services if landlords or officials are overly zealous in checking immigration status, and it contributes to an overall sense of being unwelcomed.

Public attitudes towards migrant nurses can be ambivalent. On one hand, there is high reliance on overseas staff to fill NHS shortages (the United Kingdom has a 29,000-nurse shortfall [86]) and during the COVID-19 pandemic the public lauded frontline health workers (many of whom were IENs). On the other hand, anti-immigration sentiment and rhetoric around 'taking back control' of borders created uncertainty. A stark example was the exodus of EU-trained nurses after the Brexit referendum, when new EU nurse registrations dropped by 89% in the year after 2016 [84]. Many EU nurses cited feeling unwelcomed and worried about their future rights in the United Kingdom [87]. This contraction in the European nursing workforce made the NHS even more dependent on recruitment from outside Europe.

Internationally educated nurses (IENs) in the United Kingdom report systemic barriers and bias, with many fearing repercussions if they speak up about workplace discrimination or safety concerns [88]. In 2023, charity brap found that while 75% of UK-trained NHS staff had raised racism concerns, only just over 50% of international staff had done so. Many IENs worry that complaints could mark them as 'troublemakers' or even jeopardise their job and visa [89].

Racial discrimination and microaggressions remain widespread, with IENs facing extra scrutiny, doubts about their skills and derogatory comments from colleagues and patients [89]. Some endure unfair treatment quietly, fearing that objecting could lead to accusations of arrogance [89]. Government policies further burden migrant nurses; for example, until 2020 they had to pay the Immigration Health Surcharge (IHS) to access NHS services. Though this charge was scrapped for health visa holders, other restrictions persist. Most IENs on work visas have 'no recourse to public funds' (NRPF), preventing access to state benefits and financial support [90].

A Royal College of Nursing (RCN) survey in 2024 found that international nurses were twice as likely as UK colleagues to face financial hardship, with two-thirds considering leaving the United Kingdom due to economic pressures [90]. Despite paying taxes, IENs are ineligible for benefits like Universal Credit and child support. Indefinite Leave to Remain, which removes the NRPF condition, requires 5 years of residency and costs nearly £3000, trapping many nurses in precarious circumstances. RCN leadership has warned that pushing migrant nurses into poverty could drive them away, calling for policies that treat them equitably alongside UK-born staff [90].

It is clear that the United Kingdom's immigration environment exacerbates IENs' experiences of discrimination and economic hardship, reinforcing alienation. Professional bodies and diaspora networks increasingly advocate for a more supportive system that recognises overseas nurses' vital contributions and ensures fair treatment within the NHS.

Surprisingly, there have been a handful of studies which have explored the lived experience of internationally educated nurses coming to the United Kingdom [91]. The majority of the published literature in this area comes from Norway, Finland and Canada. Ugiagbe [92] studied the integration of IENs with Nigerian heritage into the United Kingdom. She found that integration was a complex phenomenon shaped in part by challenges including immigration processes and employer practices. The participants reported personal and social integration issues alongside the issue of being accepted in the workplace. Following an initial transition phase nurses reported obstacles to career progression and discrimination.

Alexis [93] detailed a journey which probably resonates with many IENs coming to UK hospitals. This involves a transition from leaving the familiar world of their homeland to entering an unfamiliar world. Participants then describe encountering marginalisation and experiencing inequality before learning to survive and adapt to a new world. Participants described coming up against barriers which could have been avoided by host organisations as well as getting support from other IENs. This study is similar to the descriptions of coming to the United Kingdom from the Windrush generation in the 1950s [94].

Experiencing discrimination was a common theme from studies [95–97]; this was especially predominant amongst nurses from African countries but not exclusively. Such discrimination came from colleagues in the NHS as well as from patients, relatives and members of the public. In addition, many studies mention 'culture shock' when they arrive in an unfamiliar country for the first time. Despite the English language requirements some IENs report having particular difficulties with local accents and dialects [98].

Different scope of practice and ways of operating [99] presented their own challenges for IENs who had to get used to new procedures and a very different level of autonomy. There were also reported differences in the decision-making ability of UK nurses when compared to other countries [97].

Alexis [100] surveyed IENs working in NHS hospitals and found that nurses from Africa experienced the most discrimination from colleagues and patients and their relatives. While nurses from India and the Philippines reported feeling supported, nurses from Africa reported lower levels of support and assistance from white British nurses. The study recognised the difficulty some IENs experienced when trying to adapt to the culture and norms of UK society and healthcare.

Healthcare Context

The UK nursing workforce is diverse with a wide range of specialisms and advanced nursing practice roles. Unlike many other European countries, the United Kingdom differentiates its initial registration into four fields of practice. These are adult nursing, children's nursing, learning disabilities and mental health nursing [101]. This differentiation at pre-registration level is unusual and can make the placement of internationally educated nurses into anything other than adult nursing difficult. Unlike in some other countries [102] midwifery is a separate profession and it is possible to be educated as a midwife without being a registered nurse. It is possible for internationally educated midwives to undertake a specific test of competence to enter Part 2 of the NMC register [103].

Further specialisation after registration is commonplace with nurses deciding to specialise in acute hospital care, rehabilitation, critical care, oncology and a whole host of other roles. Some specialisations require specific qualifications at postgraduate level while others might be acquired through experience. The UK system also has a well-developed system of advanced nursing practice. This includes Advanced Nurse Practitioners (ANPs), often referred to by their multiprofessional title of Advanced Clinical Practitioners (ACPs), and Clinical Nurse Specialists. These individuals have advanced postgraduate qualifications which enable them to assess patients, diagnose problems and prescribe medicines [104]. As the United Kingdom does not have registration for advanced nursing practice this prevents ANPs from other countries from taking up such roles in the United Kingdom as there is no specific standard to judge competence against [105].

Specialisation is also evident in community health services where the United Kingdom has some of the widest differentiation of roles to ensure comprehensive and universal coverage for the population. Mainstream roles such as district nursing, general practice nursing, health visiting and school nursing require specialist regulated qualifications. These range from the Specialist Community Public Health Nursing (SCPHN) roles in health visiting, school nursing, occupational health nursing and sexual health nursing through to Specialist Practitioner Qualifications (SPQs) across six specialist fields of practice. The Queen's Institute of Community Nursing [106] has identified nine fields of specialist community practice including homeless and inclusion health, criminal justice nursing and palliative and end-of-life care.

Healthcare in the United Kingdom is also highly differentiated into specialisms and there is considerable task shifting between medicine and nursing and also within individual professions [107]. This means that internationally educated nurses would need to have skills in individual procedures which might not be tested through the NMC's test of competence. Many internationally educated nurses have these skills but the risk-averse nature of UK healthcare means employers would wish to retrain and assess individuals before they were allowed to practise things such as intravenous drug administration.

Nursing in the United Kingdom is made up of a workforce consisting of a range of registered practitioners and unregistered staff working as healthcare assistants or auxiliary nurses. In 2017, in England, the Nursing Associate role was introduced; this is a 2-year qualification enabling individuals to register with the NMC as a Nursing Associate. Nursing Associates were originally intended to support Registered Nurses with care delivery; they specifically are not educated to assess patients or to evaluate care [108]. The role is controversial because of issues around the scope of practice and deployment [109]. There are concerns that employers using Nursing Associates as substitutes for Registered Nurses and that as a result practitioners are exploited [110, 111].

Emigration of UK-educated nurses to other countries was at its peak between 1989 and 1990 with around 8500 nurses leaving, most commonly for Australia and Canada [112]. It dipped significantly in the intervening years but rose again from 2020. More recently the number of registered nurses applying for documentation to register abroad reached 12,000 requests on 2022/23 [113]. According to the Royal College of Nursing [66], this was associated with low salaries and workplace stress and pressure.

UK nursing qualifications were once highly regarded globally where the State Registered Nurse (SRN) or Registered General Nurse (RGN) qualification would enable registration in several other countries [113]. The current registered nurse qualifications are no longer universally regarded and UK-educated nurses seeking employment in other countries may need to pass entrance examinations [90]. Furthermore, qualifications such as Registered Nurse Mental Health (RNMH) and Registered Sick Children's Nurse (RSCN) were less universally accepted as not every country has specialisation at the point of registration [90].

Registration (Licensure) of Internationally Educated Nurses

In 2013, the Nursing and Midwifery Council decided to revise its overseas registration policy to ensure public protection and to provide a more robust assessment of nurses seeking UK registration [114]. In 2024 the NMC replaced the Overseas Adaptation Programme with a test of competence made up of two parts. Part 1 is a computer-based test (CBT) using 120 multiple choice questions while Part 2 is an Objective Structured Clinical Examination (OSCE). The OSCE consists of ten stations with four scenario-based stations designed to test assessment, planning, implementation and evaluation alongside two linked skills stations and two written stations. All ten stations must be passed and the cost of the OSCE assessment is currently £794 with a resit fee (for seven or fewer stations) of £397. The current first-time mean pass rate is 42.6% with a resit mean pass rate of 82% [115].

Prior to undertaking Part 2 of the test of competence, prospective registrants must successfully pass the CBT. The pass mark is set through a standard setting process considering the question difficulty. The CBT is provided for the NMC by Pearson VUE who have test centres in most countries around the world [116].

In addition to the test of competence, candidates seeking UK registration must demonstrate proficiency in English (speaking, reading, writing and understanding) in accordance with Schedule 4 of the Nursing and Midwifery Order 2001 [117].

The review of the Overseas Adaptation Programme was in part triggered by the high-profile Stepping Hill Hospital poisoning incidents, in 2011, for which Victorino Chua was sentenced to life imprisonment following two murders and 20 other poisoning incidents [118]. An investigation by the British Broadcasting Corporation (BBC) revealed that Victorino Chua had fraudulently represented his nursing qualifications to the NMC to gain entry to the register [119]. However, earlier Overseas Adaptation Programme issues had been raised because of fraudulent activity arising from the 'Mornington Hall' nursing home [120]. The wholesale changes to the Overseas Adaptation Programme appear to be completely disproportionate to the issues which triggered the review. The new test of competence would do little to prevent another serial killer and as we will see shortly, they have done little to prevent widespread fraud.

The move towards a test of competence have raised issues around parity for internationally educated nurses when compared with UK-educated nurses. The test of competence has been perceived as racist as it holds internationally educated nurses to a higher standard than those educated in the United Kingdom who do not need to pass a nationally mandated test. In addition, language tests have been described as structurally racist as they disadvantage internationally educated nurses from non-European Union and non-white countries [121].

Significant concerns have been raised for several years about the English language requirements and specific tests employed in assessing this. These concerns are that the scores required are exceptionally high, e.g. 7.0 in all areas for the International English Language Testing System (IELTS). Yet HCL Workforce Solutions [122] has identified that most native English speakers would only score on average 6.9. The ILETS test is also not focused on the language required to function in a healthcare setting [121]. The NMC moved to the Occupational English Test alongside ILETS in 2023 but despite this there are concerns that neither test supports integration of internationally educated nurses into the workplace and that communication and cultural differences present several challenges [123].

The test of competence may also be flawed because it makes several assumptions. Firstly, it assumes that competence is stable over time and that individuals are not able to just perform well on a single occasion [124]. Secondly, the assessment of competence often oversimplifies activities and overlooks the importance of broader knowledge and skills used in clinical reasoning and critical thinking [125]. Thirdly, candidates are confused as to why the test of competence OSCE elements differ from 'real life' performance in the NHS [126]. The final criticism of the test of competence relates to the pass criteria for the OSCE elements. It is widely accepted that healthcare is not error free [127] and what we should be aiming for is error minimisation and early identification of problems so that corrective action can be taken [128]. The OSCE assumes that people can practise perfectly all the time rather than getting them to identify errors, near misses and areas for improvement [129]. There are also concerns about failure for arbitrary issues and simply running out of time [126].

Recently there have been reports of widespread fraud at a CBT test centre run on behalf of the NMC by Pearson VUE. The Yunnik test centre in Nigeria has been responsible for widespread fraudulent activity with 'ghosting' of candidates. This is where the candidate is replaced for the test by another person. This has affected the test results of more than 500 overseas applicants calling into question their registration or preventing them moving to the second part of the test of competence [130]. A total of 48 registrants were subject to fraudulent entry proceedings [131].

Integration

IEN Profile

Internationally educated nurses (IENs) have been integral to the United Kingdom's healthcare system since the inception of the National Health Service (NHS) in 1948. From the mid-twentieth-century recruitment of Caribbean nurses in the Windrush era to today's diverse influx from Asia, Africa and Europe, the NHS in all four UK nations has long relied on overseas talent. In recent years this reliance has only grown. In the United Kingdom, nearly one-quarter of all registered nurses and midwives were trained overseas [132]. Moreover, about half of new nurse registrants each year have been educated outside the United Kingdom, the highest share in decades. As outlined earlier this trend reflects aggressive international recruitment to address domestic workforce shortages. For instance, as of 2023–2024, approximately one in six NHS staff overall report a non-British nationality, and roughly one in four NHS nurses are internationally educated, underscoring the critical contribution of IENs across the country [133].

The types and origins of IENs in the NHS are extremely diverse, spanning over 90 countries. Historically, substantial numbers came from Commonwealth nations such as India, the Philippines, Nigeria and various African and Caribbean countries. Recent data and surveys indicate that the largest groups of new international nurses in the United Kingdom come from countries like the Philippines (about 23% of recent IEN arrivals), India (22%) and Nigeria (15%), with notable cohorts also from Ghana, various East African and South Asian countries and some from Europe [132]. This multicultural workforce brings a wealth of knowledge and experience to UK health services. Many IENs arrive with strong clinical backgrounds, having practised in advanced health systems or in senior roles abroad, and they often possess unique cultural and linguistic skills. Their contribution is evident in staffing essential services and filling gaps in specialties suffering domestic shortages. Quite simply, modern NHS services cannot run without these dedicated colleagues from across the globe. The presence of IENs has also improved the cultural competence of care delivery, as nurses from diaspora communities can help bridge language and cultural barriers with patients [132]. The profile of IENs in the United Kingdom today is one of a highly skilled, internationally diverse group that is indispensable to sustaining the healthcare workforce.

Yet, despite their importance, the make-up of the international nursing cohort is continuously evolving. Policy changes (like Brexit ending EU free movement) and global trends influence the source countries; for example, since 2021 the proportion of EU-trained nurses joining the United Kingdom has declined, while recruits from countries such as Nepal and various African nations have increased [134]. All UK countries share similar challenges and opportunities in integrating these nurses, although England, by virtue of its size, hosts the majority of IENs. Each of the nation's four health services (Northern Ireland, Scotland, Wales and England) has strategies to attract and retain international staff. For instance, NHS Scotland recently launched an international recruitment hub and funded the hiring of hundreds of overseas nurses [135]. Wales and Northern Ireland have likewise welcomed nurses from abroad under targeted schemes. In England, NHS trusts have actively recruited thousands of nurses from countries including India, the Philippines, Nigeria and beyond, often through international recruitment campaigns supported and driven by NHS England policies [132].

Many internationally educated nurses (IENs) arrive in the United Kingdom with extensive experience and specialised skills, yet they often face deskilling upon entering NHS roles [136]. Surveys show that 78% of new IENs had over 5 years of experience before migrating, with nearly half exceeding a decade [132]. Despite this, most are placed in Band 5 staff nurse roles regardless of their expertise, leading to frustration over unrecognised specialisation [137]. The Royal College of Nursing (RCN) notes that international nurses are frequently assigned to junior roles that do not reflect their qualifications [132].

This lack of recognition forces many IENs into jobs they feel overqualified for. In an RCN survey, 34% of respondents said their qualifications were disregarded when applying for NHS roles [138]. Personal accounts describe nurses with advanced training working as healthcare assistants due to unacknowledged specialisation. Research by the University of Huddersfield found that IENs struggle to progress beyond Band 5 compared to UK-trained nurses [139].

Barriers to career advancement include gaps between international training and UK requirements, structural biases and limited mentorship opportunities. NHS workplace culture often assumes that IENs need prolonged adjustment periods before taking senior roles, leading to an underutilisation of skills [89]. This talent mismatch discourages long-term retention, with many IENs leaving the United Kingdom due to lack of career progression [132].

Efforts to address this issue include improved recognition of overseas qualifications by employers, bridging programmes for specialist roles and national initiatives such as the NHS Long Term Workforce Plan advocating clearer career pathways for IENs [18, 140]. The RCN urges support for IENs to work at their full skill level rather than being confined to lower-band roles [132]. Overcoming these barriers is crucial to both enhancing IEN job satisfaction and fully leveraging their expertise within the NHS workforce.

Workplace Experience

Internationally educated nurses (IENs) in the United Kingdom face significant career progression barriers, often linked to systemic racism and bias. NHS workforce data, including the Workforce Race Equality Standard (WRES), consistently shows racial and ethnic disparities, with Black and minority ethnic staff under-represented in senior roles and reporting poorer workplace treatment [64]. Despite their contributions, diaspora nurses are significantly under-represented in leadership positions, as noted by the Chief Nursing Officer of Wales [133].

Racism, both overt and subtle, impacts promotion opportunities. In a 2023 RCN survey, 46% of IENs reported experiencing racism at work and 64% felt they had been treated unfairly [138]. Black African and Caribbean nurses reported the highest levels of racist treatment (60%). NHS Staff Survey data confirms rising reports of discrimination affecting minority staff [141]. Many IENs experience shock and distress upon encountering racism, which can hinder their confidence and career prospects [142].

IENs remain clustered in Band 5 roles longer than UK-born peers, with only 49% believing they have equal access to career progression [132]. Bias in recruitment sees white British candidates more readily identified as 'management material' [121]. NHS recruitment data indicates that white applicants are more likely to be appointed than minority candidates, perpetuating under-representation in senior nursing roles. The RCN's 2025 report highlighted structural racism as a major barrier to IEN advancement, calling for employer action [132].

Workplace racism and bullying further discourage career progression. Over half (51%) of surveyed IENs reported harassment or abuse at work, including being mocked for accents or cultural references [132]. These hostile experiences impact mental health and deter nurses from seeking promotions or additional training. Some IENs, particularly those facing severe discrimination, consider leaving the United Kingdom altogether [132].

While many IENs have positive workplace experiences, systemic barriers persist. Efforts such as the NHS WRES and leadership programmes for Black, Asian and Minority Ethnic (BAME) staff aim to improve representation [143]. Employers are encouraged to enforce zero-tolerance policies on racism and ensure fairness in promotions. The NMC's diaspora forums offer a platform for addressing these challenges. Systemic racism remains a key obstacle to IEN career advancement and integration within the NHS.

The integration of internationally educated nurses (IENs) in the United Kingdom relies on active support from healthcare organisations, regulators and professional bodies [144]. NHS England has prioritised international nurse well-being, collaborating with diaspora groups to offer guidance, mentorship and networking [145]. It has also introduced standards like the 'Pastoral Care Quality Award' to encourage NHS Trusts to provide high-quality support for overseas recruits.

Regulatory bodies such as the Nursing and Midwifery Council (NMC) also play a crucial role. In 2024, the NMC established the International and Diaspora Nursing and Midwifery Associations (IDNMA) Forum to engage directly with IENs and diaspora organisations, informing policies and removing barriers in registration and career development [146]. The forum addresses issues such as discrimination and workplace inequality, shifting towards a more supportive regulatory stance [126]. Although the regulator has also come under fire for racism and cultural problems.

Professional associations and unions advocate for IENs through lobbying efforts. The Royal College of Nursing (RCN) has pushed for policy changes, such as eliminating unfair immigration rules and enforcing ethical recruitment standards outlined in the 2023 Code of Practice [132, 147]. The RCN and other bodies like Unison and the Royal College of Midwives provide networking, mentorship and guidance for overseas nurses.

At the employer level, NHS Trusts play a key role in integration, with successful organisations offering comprehensive onboarding programmes, including transitional accommodation, shadow shifts and tailored induction processes [132, 140]. NHS Employers publishes an International Recruitment Toolkit detailing best practices for supporting overseas recruits [148].

The Tropical Health and Education Trust (THET), now Global Health Partnerships, has encouraged leveraging diaspora health professionals for leadership and global health initiatives [149]. Effective integration requires long-term organisational commitment, ensuring fairness, onboarding resources and accountability, regardless of government policy changes affecting immigration and inclusion.

Community

Diaspora Nursing and Midwifery Associations in the United Kingdom play a crucial role in supporting internationally educated nurses (IENs) through professional and personal challenges. These community-led groups, such as the Philippine Nurses Association of UK and British Indian Nurses Association, serve as peer support systems that complement formal NHS induction programmes [145, 150]. They foster cultural familiarity, help newcomers navigate workplace integration and even enhance broader understanding among UK-trained nurses.

A key function of these associations is pastoral care, providing IENs with a sense of community and reducing isolation through social events, faith-based support and peer mentoring. The Nursing and Midwifery Council (NMC) acknowledges their importance in promoting well-being [146]. For example, the Filipino Nurses Association UK hosts workshops on adapting to NHS terminology while the Association of Nigerian Nurses UK celebrates cultural heritage through events like Nigerian Independence Day.

Beyond social support, diaspora groups assist with career development, offering OSCE coaching and professional mentoring. The Association of South Asian Midwives (ASAM) has helped members gain confidence and advance in their careers [146]. Some associations collaborate with NHS Trusts to provide culturally tailored induction programmes for new recruits.

Advocacy is another vital function as these groups lobby for improved conditions for international staff. Some have campaigned against costly visa and NHS surcharge fees, highlighting their impact on staff retention [151]. Policymakers, including NHS England and the NMC's IDNMA Forum, now consult with diaspora associations to shape integration policies [146]. They act as bridges between frontline nurses and system leadership, ensuring real-world concerns are addressed.

Despite their contributions, many diaspora organisations operate on limited resources. NHS England has provided funding to support their work but ongoing financial uncertainty threatens their sustainability [150, 151]. These associations transform diversity into strength, fostering belonging, professional growth and retention. Their partnership with formal institutions is key to ensuring successful NHS workforce integration.

Workplace Integration

The integration of internationally educated nurses into the NHS is shaped by their workplace experiences. While many find their work fulfilling, they also face challenges such as high workloads and staffing shortages. In a 2023 survey, 48% rated NHS staffing levels as 'poor' or 'very poor' and 45% found workloads difficult [138]. Many were surprised by the severity of these challenges, with over half reporting that staffing shortages were worse than expected (53%) and their workload heavier than anticipated (49%).

Cultural and clinical practice differences also affect integration, requiring adaptation to NHS protocols, technology and medication differences [152, 153]. Linguistic and cultural adjustments, including understanding British politeness, indirect feedback and colloquialisms, can be difficult. Miscommunication is common, leading some Trusts to implement buddy systems and diaspora groups to offer 'hospital English' lessons [91]. Over time, most IENs develop strong linguistic and cultural competence [154].

Team inclusion is crucial. While many IENs report positive experiences, others feel excluded or undervalued. Some experience 'othering', where their clinical judgement is questioned, affecting confidence [132, 154]. One IEN emphasised that UK staff must recognise their expertise despite differing training environments [132]. Successful integration requires mutual adjustment from both IENs and their teams.

Personal challenges also impact workplace performance, including financial struggles, housing difficulties and family separation [153]. Only 40% of surveyed IENs found improved work–life balance and just 39% felt financially better off in the United Kingdom [132]. Some regret their decision to migrate realising the NHS's demands outweigh expected benefits.

Despite obstacles, many IENs thrive advancing to senior roles and mentoring newcomers. The NHS benefits from their contributions, particularly in understaffed sectors like care homes and mental health services [155–157]. Patients often appreciate their compassionate care. Ultimately, workplace support, adequate staffing, cultural inclusion and fair treatment are essential for successful integration benefiting both IENs and the NHS as a whole.

Future Directions and Challenges

The title of this chapter asks if after 90 years the United Kingdom has really learnt anything about nurse migration. We can see from the arguments presented that many of the fundamental issues about migration, racism and barriers to promotion continue. Despite 90 years of experience the United Kingdom is behind other countries in recognising that IENs have saved our NHS not for the first time since its foundation in 1948. The Royal College of Nursing [132] report *Unreciprocated Care* contains a quotation from an IEN which perfectly sums up the problem. The nurse says *'I love living in the UK. I love the people. I love my job and my department. I always try to defend it to my other international nurse friends that have moved to the US, Canada or Australia. But somehow, it's too tiring to defend this country when it's not reciprocating you the care and support that we as immigrants deserve. I wish that the UK government will try to make more effort so international nurses choose to come here instead and stay'* [132], p. 6).

To some extent, tackling the barriers for IENs is just a matter of common sense and recognising that individuals who answer the call to come and support our public services should be supported to not only enter the United Kingdom but to live here with their families and access services. These individuals are not the same as economic migrants coming to the United Kingdom to seek work or refugees or asylum seekers. That is not to say that those individuals should have no right of entry but they are different to the people we invite to support our public services.

The Royal College of Nursing [132] surveyed 3000 internationally educated nurses and interviewed in depth 25 people. They found that only one-third of respondents planned to stay in the United Kingdom longer term and that two-thirds of respondents had experienced racism. The Royal College of Nursing calls for an overhaul of the immigration system for nurses with fees for visas being lowered to what they actually cost to process. Nurses working in the United Kingdom should have recourse to public funds for childcare, etc. after all they are contributing through taxation and paying National Insurance.

Racism in the UK health service remains an issue [158] and can only be tackled through active anti-racist policies which serve to protect employees through staff training, dealing appropriately with breaches of policy and rooting out structural racism at all levels [159].

Promoting Integration

Internationally there is evidence that buddying and mentoring schemes can assist with integration of IENs [113]. Of course, such schemes need to be culturally appropriate because as source countries change it may not always be possible to buddy up IENs from the same country. In addition, some specialisms such as community nursing have seen less international recruitment and therefore the availability of buddies and role models is likely to be more limited. In addition, it is important UK-educated nurses receive education about cultural differences, customs and practices to ensure that IENs are made more welcome and that colleagues have a greater understanding of how they might need support to integrate into UK teams.

Any mentoring or preceptorship period would need to be tailored to suit IENs, many of whom have considerable experience. Simply, treating IENs the same as newly qualified nurses in the United Kingdom would not work as it would lead to individuals feeling devalued and deskilled [160]. There are numerous examples of where this occurs but none as stark as Dr. Alegado who is a senior academic at the University of Worcester [161]. Having worked as an academic in China and Australia, Dr. Alegado came to the United Kingdom with a PhD and academic track record but had to return to practice as a theatre practitioner and start again on the road to becoming a nursing academic. This failure to recognise prior experience and qualifications remains an unresolved problem for IENs.

Bardi [162] suggests that integration could be improved through enhanced recruitment practices which are designed to smooth the transition to the United Kingdom and to a role in the NHS and by better preparing the existing workforce to receive IENs. This preparation should include training to develop cultural competence in order to understand people's backgrounds, experience and their home health service.

Initiatives such as the NHS Stay and Thrive initiative provide structured support to IENs to build a sense of belonging as well as maximising personal and professional growth [163]. Stay and Thrive starts pre-arrival with the provision of welcome information and assistance to relocate and settle in. It includes meeting new arrivals at the airport and supporting them to settle into their accommodation as a cohort. Ongoing support is provided to prepare IENs for their NMC test of competence assessments. Beyond this initial support, IENs get buddying, mentoring and career support to help them thrive in the UK NHS. The results show greater retention of IENs and stronger job satisfaction [164].

Mentoring, Qualifications and Promotion Opportunities

Internationally educated nurses (IENs) in the NHS face persistent barriers to role extension and career progression due to the absence of reciprocity in recognising skills across organisations [160]. Despite attempts to address this, progress has been slow [165], and even enhanced care practitioners do not automatically receive an extended scope of practice when moving between organisations.

Supporting IENs in gaining additional qualifications is crucial but managers and educators must acknowledge culturally different approaches to learning [160].

Systems recognising prior formal and experiential learning should be implemented to prevent unnecessary repetition of courses.

Promotion barriers remain significant with IENs often feeling that career advancement depends on being 'in the right place at the right time' [160], p. 65. Structural and language obstacles hinder their ability to apply for senior roles [166], though some NHS organisations now offer workshops to assist IENs in career planning [148]. A survey of Filipino nurses in the United Kingdom found that out of 22,000 registered nurses educated in the Philippines, only 19 had attained senior management salaries under the Agenda for Change pay system [167].

Advanced Practice Nursing (APN) in the United Kingdom is currently unregulated, leaving IENs with APN qualifications unrecognised [168]. The Florence Nightingale Foundation found that many IENs possess APN attributes but cannot receive formal recognition. As the Nursing and Midwifery Council (NMC) moves towards APN regulation, it is likely to introduce a portfolio route which must accommodate IENs to ensure equal recognition.

Diaspora associations have established mentoring programmes to support IENs in achieving promotion. The Filipino Nurses Association UK offers 6-month mentoring by senior nurses, including the Chief Nursing Officer for England [169]. While formally unevaluated, this initiative may have contributed to several IENs advancing to Chief Nurse and Nurse Director positions in recent years, creating role models to help others ascend to senior NHS roles.

Conclusion

This comprehensive analysis highlights the critical role that internationally educated nurses (IENs) play in sustaining the United Kingdom's healthcare workforce, amid ongoing domestic shortages and persistent structural challenges. While the NHS continues to rely heavily on international recruitment to address staffing gaps, this strategy is fraught with ethical dilemmas, particularly around recruitment from WHO red list countries. Simultaneously, domestic workforce planning has suffered from underinvestment, inconsistent policy and inadequate retention strategies, particularly for early-career nurses. There has been a lack of learning from previous international recruitment efforts and the United Kingdom consistently makes the same mistakes making nurses who migrate to the United Kingdom feel unwelcome, disadvantaged and subject to abuse.

It is clear that IENs often face significant barriers upon arrival, including complex regulatory requirements, financial burdens and the broader societal implications of the United Kingdom's hostile immigration environment. These challenges are compounded by systemic racism and unequal access to career progression, despite the indispensable contributions of IENs to patient care and service continuity.

To ensure a sustainable and ethically sound nursing workforce, the United Kingdom must commit to long-term, fully funded workforce planning that prioritises training, retention and support for both domestic and internationally educated nurses. Simultaneously, immigration policies must be reformed to foster inclusion and stability for those who choose to serve in the NHS. The NHS also needs to get to grips with racism and a wider cultural issues which leave nurses feeling unsupported. Without such reforms, the United Kingdom risks further exacerbating health inequalities and undermining the very system that depends so heavily on the compassion, skill and resilience of its diverse nursing workforce.

References

1. Nursing and Midwifery Council. Nursing and midwifery register grows but pace of international nurse recruitment slows. NMC: London; 2024. [cited 07.04.2025] Available from https://www.nmc.org.uk/news/news-and-updates/nursing-and-midwifery-register-grows-but-pace-of-international-nurse-recruitment-slows/
2. My Healthcare Recruit. UK October 2024 Budget: implications for NHS trusts and International Recruitment. Blog 28 November 2024. [cited 07.04.2025] Available from https://myhealthcarerecruit.com/2024/11/28/uk-october-2024-budget-implications-for-nhs-trusts-and-international-recruitment/
3. World Health Organization. WHO health workforce support and safeguards list 2023. Geneva: WHO; 2023.
4. Nursing and Midwifery Council. The NMC register UK mid-year update; 2024 NMC: London.
5. NHS Digital. NHS Vacancy Statistics, England, April 2015–December 2024; 2025, NHSE: London.
6. Royal College of Nursing. The nursing workforce in Scotland; 2024, RCN: Edinburgh.
7. Welsh Government. NHS vacancy statistics; 2024, Welsh Government: Cardiff.
8. Royal College of Nursing. Northern Ireland fair pay and safe staffing campaign; 2024, RCN: Belfast.
9. Birch S. Demand-based models and market failure in health care: projecting shortages and surpluses in doctors and nurses. Health Econ Policy Law. 2019;14(2):291–4. https://doi.org/10.1017/S1744133118000336.
10. The King's Fund. Activity in the NHS; 2024, The King's Fund: London.
11. Imison C, Castle-Clarke S, Watson R. Reshaping the workforce to deliver the care patients need 2016, Research Report. Nuffield Trust: London.
12. Sansum J, Tucker A. Is the left shift impossible? 2015 [cited 16.04.2025] NHS Confederation: London. Available from https://www.nhsconfed.org/long-reads/left-shift-mission-impossible
13. Palmer B. Doing right when you are wrong: perspectives on workforce planning in the NHS in uncertain times; 2022 [cited 16.04.2025] Blog Nuffield Trust: London. Available from https://www.nuffieldtrust.org.uk/news-item/doing-right-when-you-are-wrong-perspectives-on-workforce-planning-in-the-nhs-in-uncertain-times
14. Buchan J, Edwards N. Nursing numbers in Britain: the argument for workforce planning. BMJ. 2000;320(7241):1067–70. https://doi.org/10.1136/bmj.320.7241.1067.
15. Jones K, Weatherly H, Birch S et al. Unit costs for health and social care 2022 manual; 2022, University of Kent: Canterbury.
16. Thompson F, Hodge G, Edge D, Howes S, Jamison C, Fisher M, Jones A. Understanding the risk factors for student attrition across pre-registration nursing and midwifery programmes in a United Kingdom university: a sequential explanatory mixed methods study. Nurse Educ Today. 2025;145:106503. https://doi.org/10.1016/j.nedt.2024.106503.
17. RCN. Royal College of Nursing Huge increase in nurses quitting early in 'perfect storm' for patient care, as RCN warns NHS reforms at risk; 2024. RCN: London.
18. NHS England. NHS long term workforce plan. London: NHSE; 2023.
19. Royal College of Physicians. RCP responds to news that revised NHS England Long Term Workforce Plan will be published in 2025. London: RCP; 2024.

20. Council of Deans for Health. Briefing: UCAS deadline applicant statistics for January 2024. London: CoDH; 2024.
21. UCAS. Nursing applications soar as UCAS publishes latest undergraduate applicant analysis. London: University and College Admissions Services; 2021.
22. Murphy R. What possible reason could there be for nursing applications to have fallen? 2024, Funding the Future: Cambridge. [cited 16.04.2025] Available from https://www.taxresearch.org.uk/Blog/2024/02/15/what-possible-reason-could-there-be-for-nursing-applications-to-have-fallen/
23. The Health Foundation. Change in the profile of nursing students from England. London: The Health Foundation; 2017.
24. Royal College of Nursing. 2023 nursing in numbers. London: RCN; 2023.
25. Heaslip V, Board M, Duckworth V, Thomas L. Widening participation in nurse education: an integrative literature review. Nurse Educ Today. 2017;59:66–74. https://doi.org/10.1016/j.nedt.2017.08.016.
26. McAnea C. Removal of the nursing student bursary is a reckless experiment; 2017, [cited 16.04.2025] Health Services Journal, available from https://www.hsj.co.uk/workforce/removal-of-the-nursing-student-bursary-is-a-reckless-experiment/7016483.article
27. Scammell J. The implications of nurse shortages. Br J Nurs. 2019;28(3):208.
28. Ford S. Nursing degree applicants fall 23% in wake of bursary loss; 2017, Nursing Times Online. 2 Feb 2017 [cited 16.04.2025] Available from https://www.nursingtimes.net/education-and-training/nursing-degree-applicants-fall-23-in-wake-of-bursary-loss-02-02-2017/#:~:text=02%20February%2C%202017%20By%20Steve,had%20fallen%20by%20around%2020%25
29. Buchan J, Ball J, Shembavnekar N, Charlesworth A. Building the NHS nursing workforce in England. The Health Foundation: London; 2020.
30. Launder M. Student nurses to receive living cost grant from September 2020; 2019, Nursing in Practice [cited 16.04.2025] available from https://www.nursinginpractice.com/latest-news/student-nurses-to-receive-living-cost-grants-from-september-2020/
31. Gershlick B, Charlesworth A. Health and Social care workforce: priorities for the new government. The Health Foundation: London; 2019.
32. Nursing and Midwifery Council. The NMC register 1 April 2022–31 March 2023; 2023, NMC: London.
33. Ejebu O-Z, Turnbull J, Atherton I, et al. What might make nurses stay? A protocol for discrete choice experiments to understand NHS nurses' preferences at early- career and late-career stages. BMJ Open. 2024;14:e075066. https://doi.org/10.1136/bmjopen-2023-075066.
34. Kelly E, Stoye G, Warner M. Factors associated with staff retention in the NHS acute sector. London: Institute for Fiscal Studies; 2022.
35. Buaki-Sogo MA, Goldspink S, Engward H. Workforce assets: recognising the value of long-serving nurses and midwives. Nurs Times. 2023;119:11.
36. Leary A. "Rookie factor": why healthcare workforce policy needs to embrace experience. Br Med J. 2024;387:q2836. https://doi.org/10.1136/bmj.q2836.
37. Burau V, Buch Mejsner S, Falkenbach M, et al. Post-COVID health policy responses to healthcare workforce capacities: a comparative analysis of health system resilience in six European countries. Health Policy. 2024;139:104962. https://doi.org/10.1016/j.healthpol.2023.104962.
38. Yarbrough S, Martin P, Alfred D, McNeill C. Professional values, job satisfaction, career development, and intent to stay. Nurs Ethics. 2016;24(6):675–85. https://doi.org/10.1177/0969733015623098.
39. Brook J, Aitken L, Webb R, MacLaren J, Salmon D. Characteristics of successful interventions to reduce turnover and increase retention of early career nurses: a systematic review. Int J Nurs Stud. 2019;91:47–59. https://doi.org/10.1016/j.ijnurstu.2018.11.003.
40. Cleaver K, Markowski M, Wels J. Factors influencing older nurses' decision making around the timing of retirement: an exploratory mixed-methods study. J Nurs Manag. 2022;30(1):169–78. https://doi.org/10.1111/jonm.13447.

41. Rolewicz L, Palmer B. The NHS workforce in numbers; 2019 Nuffield Trust: London [cited 16.04.2025] Available from https://www.nuffieldtrust.org.uk/resource/the-nhs-workforce-in-numbers
42. NHS Digital. Narrowing of NHS gender divide but men still the majority in senior roles; 2020. NHS Digital: London [cited 16.04.2025] Available from https://www.wired-gov.net/wg/news.nsf/articles/Narrowing+of+NHS+gender+divide+but+men+still+the+majority+in+senior+roles+08032018160500?open
43. NHS England. NHS workforce race equality standard 2023 data analysis report for NHS Trusts; 2024 [cited 16.04.2025] NHS England: London. Available from https://www.england.nhs.uk/publication/nhs-workforce-race-equality-standard-2023-data-analysis-report-for-nhs-trusts/
44. Kline R, Warmington J. Too Hot to Handle? Why concerns about racism are not heard... or acted on. BRAP: Birmingham; 2024.
45. Rafferty AM, Solano D. The rise and demise of the Colonial Nursing Service: British Nurses in the Colonies, 1896-1966. Nurs Hist Rev. 2007;15:147–54. https://doi.org/10.1891/1062-8061.15.147.
46. Solano D, Rafferty AM. Can lessons be learned from history? The origins of the British imperial nurse labour market: a discussion paper. Int J Nurs Stud. 2007;44(6):1055–63. https://doi.org/10.1016/j.ijnurstu.2006.07.004.
47. Yeates N. Migration and nursing in Ireland: an internationalist history. Trans Migration Social Change. 2009;5(1):1–20.
48. Ryan L. Who do you think you are? Irish nurses encountering ethnicity and constructing identity in Britain. Ethn Racial Stud. 2007;30(3):416–38. https://doi.org/10.1080/01419870701217498.
49. Stewart J. Angels or aliens? Refugee nurses in Britain, 1938 to 1942. Med Hist. 2003;47(2):149–72.
50. Rafferty AM, Robinson J. Nursing history and the politics of welfare. Abingdon-on-Thames: Taylor & Francis; 2005.
51. Brooks J. From "unwanted Jew" to "a brighter professional future": Kinder girls and the nursing profession in wartime Britain. JHS. 2020;51(1) https://doi.org/10.14324/111.444.jhs.2020v51.006.
52. Ali L. Caribbean Women and the NHS; 2021, Black History Month blog [cited 16.04.2025]. Available from https://www.blackhistorymonth.org.uk/article/section/nhs-and-healthcare/caribbean-women-nhs/#:~:text=From%201949%2C%20advertisements%20were%20placed%20in%20the,for%20work%20as%20auxiliaries%20and%20trainee%20nurses.&text=Trainee%20nurses%20were%20drawn%20from%20all%20over,majority%20were%20recruited%20from%20the%20Caribbean%20Islands
53. Simões R. Remembering the contribution of Windrush nurses to the NHS; 2023, Science Museum Group: London [cited 16.04.2025] Available from https://blog.sciencemuseumgroup.org.uk/remembering-the-contribution-of-windrush-nurses-to-the-nhs/
54. Batnitzky A, McDowell L. Migration, nursing, institutional discrimination and emotional/affective labour: ethnicity and labour stratification in the UK National Health Service. Soc Cult Geogr. 2011;12(2):181–201. https://doi.org/10.1080/14649365.2011.545142.
55. Olwig KF. Female immigration and the ambivalence of dirty care work: Caribbean nurses in imperial Britain. Ethnography. 2017;19(1):44–62. https://doi.org/10.1177/1466138117697744.
56. Yeo C. How did the citizenship and immigration status of the Windrush generation change over time? 2023, Blog Free Movement [cited 16.04.2025] Available from https://freemovement.org.uk/a-short-guide-to-the-legal-position-and-history-of-the-windrush-generation/
57. Serrant L. You called...and we came; 2018 [cited 16.04.2025] Available from https://lauraserrant.wordpress.com/2018/02/12/you-called-and-we-came/
58. Campbell J. Windrush scandal; 2023, EBSCO Research Starters. [cited 16.04.2025] Available from https://www.ebsco.com/research-starters/law/windrush-scandal

59. JCWI. The Joint Council for the Welfare of Immigrants, Windrush scandal explained. London: JCWI; 2024.
60. Opinion. A question of identity and equality in multicultural Britain; 2016, Opinion: London. [cited 16.04.2025] Available from https://www.opinium.com/wp-content/uploads/2016/08/a_question_of_identity_and_equality_in_multicultural_britain_0.pdf
61. Connell K. Debating the 'success' of multiculturalism misses the point – it's simply part of life in Britain today; 2023, The Conversation 3 Oct 2023. [cited 16.04.2025] Available from https://theconversation.com/debating-the-success-of-multiculturalism-misses-the-point-its-simply-part-of-life-in-britain-today-214657#:~:text=The%20picture%20today&text=In%201942%2C%20it%20was%20estimated,has%20now%20become%20irreversibly%20multicultural
62. James R. 'More diverse and culturally inclusive': post-war immigration and its impact on British culture; 2022, Blog University of Portsmouth. [cited 16.04.2025] Available from https://history.port.ac.uk/?p=2668#:~:text=Culture%20involves%20the%20characteristics%2C%20traits,cuisine%2C%20music%2C%20and%20entertainment
63. NHS England. NHS Workforce Race Equality Standard (WRES); 2015, NHSE: London [cited 16.04.2025] Available from https://www.england.nhs.uk/about/equality/equality-hub/workforce-equality-data-standards/equality-standard/
64. NHS England. NHS Workforce Race Equality Standard (WRES) 2022 data analysis report for NHS trusts; 2023, NHSE: London.
65. Cox A v NHS Commissioning Board (Operating as NHS England/NHS Improvement): 2415350/2020 and 2401365/2021. [cited 16.04.2025] Available from https://www.gov.uk/employment-tribunal-decisions/ms-a-cox-v-nhs-commissioning-board-operating-as-nhs-england-slash-nhs-improvement-2415350-slash-2020-and-2401365-slash-2021
66. Royal College of Nursing. Nursing Exodus: nurses fleeing England for better pay. London: RCN; 2024.
67. Campbell D. Thousands of foreign nurses a year leave UK to work abroad; 2024. The Guardian 25 March 2024. [cited 16.04.2025] Available from https://www.theguardian.com/society/2024/mar/25/thousands-of-foreign-nurses-a-year-leave-uk-to-work-abroad
68. Walsh PW. Policy primer: The UK's 2021 points-based immigration system. Oxford: The Migration Observatory; 2021.
69. UK Parliament. The UK's new points-based immigration system; 2022. House of Commons Library Research Briefing. UK Parliament: London.
70. Office for National Statistics. Long-term international migration, provisional: year ending June 2024. London: ONS; 2024.
71. Best for Britain. Your questions on immigration answered: What is migration? And why are some people always talking about it? 2024, [cited 16.04.2025] Available from https://www.bestforbritain.org/your_questions_on_immigration_answered
72. Refugee Council. The truth about channel crossings and the impact of the Illegal Migration Act; 2023, Refugee Council: London [cited 16.04.2025] Available from https://www-media.refugeecouncil.org.uk/media/documents/The-truth-about-channel-crossings-and-the-impact-of-the-illegal-migration-act-Oct-2023.pdf
73. Manning A. In brief... growth and immigration: unpicking the confusion; 2023, CentrePiece Spring 2023. LSE: London.
74. JCWI. The Joint Council for the Welfare of Immigrants, Making the UK a welcoming environment for all migrants. London: JCWI; 2023.
75. House of Lords. Library briefing: impact of 'Hostile Environment' 2018, Policy debate 14 June 2018. House of Lords: London.
76. Salah L. Health and care worker visa guide 2025, 2024. London: Borderless.
77. Capital Nurse International Recruitment. Managers guide for overseas nurses. London: Capital Nurse; 2022.
78. Palmer B, Leone C, Pew A, Davies M, Appleby J. Recruitment of nurses from overseas: return on investment. London: Nuffield Trust; 2021.

79. NHS Employers. Code of practice red and amber list of countries; 2025, [cited 16.04.2025] NHS Employers: London. Available from: https://www.nhsemployers.org/articles/code-practice-red-and-amber-list-countries
80. Ahmat A, et al. The health workforce status in the WHO African Region: findings of a cross-sectional study. BMJ Glob Health. 2022;7(Suppl 1):e008317. https://doi.org/10.1136/bmjgh-2021-008317.
81. Africa Europe Foundation. Health – Addressing the health workforce crisis in Africa and in Europe; 2022, [cited 16.04.2025] Available from https://www.africaeuropefoundation.org/stories/health-addressing-the-health-workforce-crisis-in-africa-and-in-europe/
82. World Health Organization. WHO Global Code of Practice on the International Recruitment of Health Personnel; 2010, Geneva: World Health Organisation. [cited 16.04.2025] Available from: https://www.who.int/publications-detail-redirect/who-global-code-of-practice-on-the-international-recruitment-of-health-personnel
83. Nursing and Midwifery Council. The NMC register: mid-year update 1 April – 30 September 2022; 2022, [cited 16.04.2025] Available from: https://www.nmc.org.uk/globalassets/sitedocuments/data-reports/sep-2022/0082a-mid-year-data-report-uk-web.pdf
84. Campbell D. NHS 'unethical' in recruiting nurses from short-staffed countries; 2023, The Guardian. [cited 16.04.2025] Available from: https://www.theguardian.com/uk-news/2023/nov/30/nhs-unethical-in-recruiting-nurses-from-short-staffed-countries
85. Qureshi A, Morris M, Mort L. Access Denied: the human impact of the hostile environment; 2020, IPPR. [cited 16.04.2025] Available from: https://www.ippr.org
86. Das S. Overseas nurses in the UK forced to pay out thousands if they want to quit jobs; 2022, The Guardian, 27 March. [cited 16.04.2025] Available from: https://www.theguardian.com
87. Campbell D. 'Brexit blamed as record number of EU nurses give up on Britain'; 2018, The Guardian, 25 April. [cited 16.04.2025] Available from: https://www.theguardian.com/society/2018/apr/25/brexit-blamed-record-number-eu-nurses-give-up-britain
88. Sobrany S. We must all help combat racism; 2023, RCN President's Blog, 21 March. [cited 16.04.2025] Available from: https://www.rcn.org.uk
89. Pressley C, Newton D, et al. Global migration and factors that support acculturation and retention of international nurses: a systematic review. Int J Nurs Stud Adv. 2022;4:100083. https://doi.org/10.1016/j.ijnsa.2022.100083.
90. Royal College of Nursing. Letter to the home secretary and secretary of state for health and social care on the visa fee increase. RCN London; 2023
91. Lanada JA, Culligan K. The experiences of internationally educated nurses who joined the nursing workforce in England. Br J Nurs. 2024;33(2):78–84. https://doi.org/10.12968/bjon.2024.33.2.78.
92. Ugiagbe IM. Integration of Internationally Educated Nurses to the UK: the Lived Experience of Nurses with Nigerian Heritage in the London Region; 2022, PhD thesis University of Middlesex: London.
93. Alexis O. 'Internationally educated nurses' experiences in a hospital in England: an exploratory study. Scand J Caring Sci. 2013;27:962–8. https://doi.org/10.1111/scs.12014.
94. Serrant L. You called and we came: remembering nurses of the Windrush generation; 2020, Black History Month. [cited 16.04.2025] Available from https://www.blackhistorymonth.org.uk/article/section/the-windrush-generation/called-came-remembering-nurses-windrush-generation/#:~:text=There%20are%20many%20stories%20of%20the%20challenges,recognition%20and%20professional%20levels%20they%20arrived%20with
95. Likupe G. Experiences of African nurses and the perception of their managers in the NHS. J Nurs Manag. 2015;23(2):231–41. https://doi.org/10.1111/jonm.12119.
96. O'Brien T, Ackroyd S. Understanding the recruitment and retention of overseas nurses: realist case study research in National Health Service Hospitals in the UK. Nurs Inq. 2012;19(1):39–50. https://doi.org/10.1111/j.1440-1800.2011.00572.x.
97. Taylor B. The experiences of overseas nurses working in the NHS: results of a qualitative study. Divers Health Soc Care. 2005;2:17–272.

98. Okougha M, Tilki M. Experience of overseas nurses: the potential for Misunderstanding. Br J Nurs. 2010;19(2):102–6. https://doi.org/10.12968/bjon.2010.19.2.46293.
99. Safari K, McKenna L, Davis J. Transition experiences of internationally qualified health care professionals: a narrative scoping review. Int J Nurs Stud. 2022;129:104221. https://doi.org/10.1016/j.ijnurstu.2022.104221.
100. Alexis O. Internationally recruited nurses' experiences in England: a survey approach. Nurs Outlook. 2014;63:238–44. https://doi.org/10.1016/j.outlook.2014.10.005.
101. Nursing and Midwifery Council. Standards of proficiency for registered nurses. London: NMC; 2018.
102. Neal S, Nove S, Bar-Zeev S, Pairman S, Ryan E, Hoope-Bender PT, Homer CSE. An analysis of the global diversity of midwifery pre-service education pathways. Women Birth. 2023;26(5):439–45. https://doi.org/10.1016/j.wombi.2023.03.002.
103. Nursing and Midwifery Council. Test of competence 2021: Midwifery test specification for candidates. London: NMC; 2023.
104. Bond C, Plotkin L, Stacey G. Consideration of the impact of additional regulation of advanced practice on internationally educated nurses and midwives working in the UK: a rapid evidence check. Florence Nightingale Foundation: London; 2024.
105. Anderson M. Advanced practice regulation needs 'accessible pathways' for international nurses; 2024, Nursing in Practice 14 November 2024. [cited 16.04.2025] Available from https://www.nursinginpractice.com/latest-news/advanced-practice-regulation-needs-accessible-pathways-for-international-nurses/#:~:text=A%20quarter%20of%20internationally%20educated%20nurses%20and,the%20UK%20felt%20hindered%20in%20accessing%20this
106. Queen's Institute of Community Nursing. Field specific standards of education and practice for community specialist practitioner qualifications. London: QICN; 2022.
107. van Schalkwyk MC, Bourek A, Kringos DS, Siciliani L, Barry MM, De Maeseneer J, McKee M. The best person (or machine) for the job: rethinking task shifting in healthcare. Health Policy. 2020;124(12):1379–86. https://doi.org/10.1016/j.healthpol.2020.08.008.
108. Royal College of Nursing. RCN position on the role and scope of practice of the Nursing Associate. London: RCN; 2024.
109. Khan A, Gurbutt R. Registered nurses' perceptions of nursing associates' professional identity; 2024. Br J Nurs. 33(15):713–7. https://doi.org/10.12968/bjon.2024.0054.
110. Dean E. Nursing associates: NHS success story or a staffing stop-gap? Nurs Stand. 2023;38(6):26–9. https://doi.org/10.7748/ns.38.6.26.s14.
111. Queen's Institute of Community Nursing. Position statement: nursing associates in community nursing settings. London: QICN; 2024.
112. Buchan J, Seccombe I, Thomas S. Overseas mobility of UK based nurses. Int J Nurs Stud. 1997;34(1):54–62. https://doi.org/10.1016/S0020-7489(96)00015-6.
113. Bazeer N, Kelly E, Buchan J. Nursing locally, thinking globally: UK-registered nurses and their intentions to leave. The Health Foundation: London; 2024.
114. Ford S. NMC asks for views on overseas nurse testing plan; 2013, Nursing Times, 09 September 2013 [cited 16.04.2025] Available from https://www.nursingtimes.net/leadership/nmc-asks-for-views-on-overseas-nurse-testing-plan-09-09-2013/
115. Nursing and Midwifery Council. Test if competence pass rates and number of candidates; 2024, NMC: London. [cited 16.04.2025] Available from https://www.nmc.org.uk/registration/joining-the-register/toc/pass-rates-and-candidate-numbers/2024/
116. Nursing and Midwifery Council. CBT – test of competence for nurses and midwives; 2024, NMC: London. [cited 16.04.2025] Available from https://www.nmc.org.uk/registration/joining-the-register/toc/toc-nursing-and-midwifery/cbt/
117. UK Parliament. The Nursing and Midwifery Order 2001; 2001, SI 2002/253.
118. Merrifield N. Stepping Hill nurse Victorino Chua given life sentence; 2015, Nursing Times, May 2015. [cited 16.04.2025] Available from https://www.nursingtimes.net/leadership/stepping-hill-nurse-victorino-chua-given-life-sentence-19-05-2015/

119. McCarthy M. Mass poisoning sparks foreign nurse checks; 2015, Sky News [cited 16.04.2025] available from https://news.sky.com/story/amp/mass-poisoning-sparks-foreign-nurses-checks-10359086
120. Oriaku R (On the Application Of) v Nursing And Midwifery Council [2017] EWHC 235 (Admin).
121. Ugiagbe IM, Liu LQ, Markowski M, Allan H. A critical race analysis of structural and institutional racism: rethinking overseas registered nurses' recruitment to and working conditions in the United Kingdom. Nurs Inq. 2023;30(1):e12512. https://doi.org/10.1111/nin.12512.
122. HCL Workforce Solutions. IELTS and declining nurse recruitment: Don't blame Brexit; 2017, HCL: London [cited 16.04.2025] Available from https://www.hclworkforce.com/wp-content/uploads/2017/05/HCL-Workforce-IELTS-Report.pdf
123. Stubbs F. Recruitment of nurses from India and their experiences of an Overseas Nurses Program. Nurs Crit Care. 2017;22(3):176–83. https://doi.org/10.1111/nicc.12181.
124. Becker H, Ndlovu C, Huang YC, Rowin T. Change over time in ratings of new nurses on the appraisal of nursing practice. J Nurs Adm. 2019;49(10):503–8. https://doi.org/10.1097/NNA.0000000000000794.
125. Fukada M. Nursing competency: definition, structure and development. Yonago Acta Med. 2018;61(1):1–7. https://doi.org/10.33160/yam.2018.03.001.
126. Davis D, Sharma S, Taylor M. Language tests and tests of competence for registration purposes – a scoping review of the experiences of overseas nurses. Contemp Nurse. 2024;60(4):420–32. https://doi.org/10.1080/10376178.2024.2318360.
127. Sameera V, Bindra A, Rath GP. Human errors and their prevention in healthcare. J Anaesthesiol Clin Pharmacol. 2021;37(3):328–35. https://doi.org/10.4103/joacp.JOACP_364_19.
128. O'Connor E, Coates HM, Yardley IE, Wu AW. Disclosure of patient safety incidents: a comprehensive review. Int J Qual Health Care. 2010;22(5):371–9. https://doi.org/10.1093/intqhc/mzq042.
129. Foster S. Are the tests for overseas nurses' fair? Br J Nurs. 2018;27(9):525. https://doi.org/10.12968/bjon.2018.27.9.525.
130. Mitchell G. Security concerns see NMC suspend testing at almost 50 centres; 2023, Nursing Times 19 July 2023 [cited 16.04.2025] Available from https://www.nursingtimes.net/professional-regulation/security-concerns-see-nmc-suspend-testing-at-almost-50-centres-19-07-2023/
131. Nursing and Midwifery Council. The action we're taking following concerns about the Yunnik test centre; 2023, NMC: London. [cited 16.04.2025] Available from https://www.nmc.org.uk/news/news-and-updates/the-action-were-taking-following-concerns-about-the-yunnik-test-centre/
132. Royal College of Nursing. Unreciprocated care: why internationally educated nursing staff are leaving the UK. London: RCN; 2025.
133. THET. Embracing opportunities to strengthen and engage diaspora contributions to the NHS; 2023, Global Health Partnerships, 29 November. [cited 16.04.2025] Available at: https://www.globalhealthpartnerships.org/embracing-opportunities-to-strengthen-and-engage-diaspora-contributions-to-the-nhs/
134. NHS Employers. International recruitment toolkit: an interactive guide to encourage and enable good practice in the NHS; 2021, London: NHS Confederation. [cited 16.04.2025] Available at: https://www.nhsemployers.org/sites/default/files/2021-07/NHS%20International%20recruitment%20toolkit%20%2828.06.21%29.pdf
135. Maclaren A, Locock L, Skea Z, Angell L, Cleland J, Dawson T, et al. 'Come and work here!' a qualitative exploration of local community-led initiatives to recruit and retain health care staff in remote and rural areas of the UK. J Health Serv Res Policy. 2025;30 https://doi.org/10.1177/13558196251318607.
136. Omiyi D, Wilkinson E, Smith B. Exploring the motivations, challenges, and integration of internationally educated healthcare workers in the UK: a scoping review. Policy Polit Nurs Pract. 2025;26(2):117–35. https://doi.org/10.1177/15271544241289605.

137. Garside J, Pressley C, Stephenson J, Newton D, Sanderson L, Duodu PA, Simkhada B, Pallam M, Gillibrand W, Internationally educated nurses experience of the first two years working and living in England: a mixed methods study; 2023, Health and Wellbeing Academy University of Huddersfield. 2023 Jun 29.
138. Royal College of Nursing. Valuing Nursing in the UK; 2023, London: Royal College of Nursing. [cited 16.04.2025] Available at: http://www.rcn.org.uk/Professional-Development/publications/valuing-nursing-in-the-uk-uk-pub-010-695
139. University of Huddersfield. Long term experiences and career progression of internationally educated nurses; 2023, Huddersfield, University of Huddersfield. [cited 16.04.2025] Available at: www.hud.ac.uk/media/assets/document/hhs/Longterm_Experiences_and_Career_Progression_Web.pdf
140. Rajpoot A, Merriman C, Rafferty AM, Henshall C. Transitioning experiences of internationally educated nurses in host countries. a narrative systematic review. Int J Nurs Stud Adv. 2024;27:100195. https://doi.org/10.1016/j.ijnsa.2024.100195.
141. NHS England. NHS Staff Survey: National Results; 2025, NHSE: London [cited 16.04.2025] Available at: http://www.nhsstaffsurveys.com/results/national-results
142. Nursing and Midwifery Council. Spotlight on Nursing and Midwifery; 2023, London, Nursing and Midwifery Council. [cited 16.04.2025] Available at: http://www.nmc.org.uk/globalassets/sitedocuments/data-reports/insight-spotlight/2023/spotlight-on-nursing-and-midwifery-report-2023.pdf
143. Adhikari R, Corcoran J, Smith P, Rodgers S, Suleiman R, Barber K. It's ok to be different: supporting black and minority ethnic nurses and midwives in their professional development in the UK; 2023. Nurse Educ Pract. 66:103508. https://doi.org/10.1016/j.nepr.2022.103508.
144. Unsworth J, Puthenpurakal A, The process of developing and implementing health and nursing policy. Implications of research and opportunities to influence. Int Nurs Rev. 2024;71(4):695–705. https://doi.org/10.1111/inr.13022.
145. NHS England. International nursing and midwifery associations; 2025, NHSE: London [cited 16.04.2025] Available at: https://www.england.nhs.uk/nursingmidwifery/international-recruitment/international-nursing-and-midwifery-associations/
146. Nursing and Midwifery Council. International and Diaspora Nursing and Midwifery Associations Forum; 2024, Nursing & Midwifery Council: London [cited 16.04.2025] Available at: https://www.nmc.org.uk/about-us/working-with-others/our-engagement-forums/inma-forum/
147. Garcia-Dia MJ. The ethical recruitment of internationally educated nurses: A leadership perspective on labor migration. Nurse Lead. 2022;20(1):43–7. https://doi.org/10.1016/j.mnl.2021.10.002.
148. Bowers B, Haq NU, Young A, Oldman C. Valuing internationally educated nurses and diversity in the community nursing workforce. Evid Based Nurs. 2024;0:1–2. https://doi.org/10.1136/ebnurs-2024-104158.
149. THET. Experts in Our Midst: recognising the contribution NHS diaspora staff make to global health; 2021, THET: London [cited 16.04.2025] Available at: https://www.globalhealthpartnerships.org/wp-content/uploads/2021/08/Experts-in-Our-Midst_2021Report.pdf
150. Puthenpurakal A. Jabali Men's Network – shaping leadership with the global majority; 2023, Evidence-Based Nursing blog, 7 May. [cited 16.04.2025] Available at: https://blogs.bmj.com/ebn/2023/05/07/jabali-mens-network-shaping-leadership-with-the-global-majority/
151. Madigan EA, McWhirter E, Westwood G, Oshikanlu R, Iregi ZM, Nyika M, Bayuo J. Nurses finding a global voice by becoming influential leaders through advocacy; 2023. Clin Integr Care. 2023;20:100165. https://doi.org/10.1016/j.intcar.2023.100165.
152. Roth C, Berger S, Krug K, Mahler C, Wensing M. Internationally trained nurses and host nurses' perceptions of safety culture, work-life-balance, burnout, and job demand during workplace integration: a cross-sectional study. BMC Nurs. 2021;20:1–5. https://doi.org/10.1186/s12912-021-00581-8.

153. Shiju M, Hall H, Lee C, Whitehouse C. Barriers and enablers of successful workplace integration of internationally educated nurses (IENs) in a host country: a qualitative evidence synthesis. Policy Polit Nurs Pract. 2024 Nov;25(4):228–40. https://doi.org/10.1177/15271544241276860.
154. Dahl K, Nortvedt L, Schrøder J, Bjørnnes AK. Internationally educated nurses and resilience: A systematic literature review. Int Nurs Rev. 2022 Sep;69(3):405–15. https://doi.org/10.1111/inr.12787.
155. Baumann A, Crea-Arsenio M, Ross D, Blythe J. Diversifying the health workforce: a mixed methods analysis of an employment integration strategy. Hum Resour Health. 2021;19(1):62. https://doi.org/10.1186/s12960-021-00606-y.
156. Lee R, Beckford D, Jakabne L, Hirst L, Cordon C, Quan S, Collins J, Baumann A, Blythe J. Multiorganizational Partnerships: A Mechanism for Increasing the Employment of Internationally Educated Nurses. Nurs Leadersh. 2021;34(3) https://doi.org/10.12927/cjnl.2021.26593.
157. Cubelo F, Parviainen A, Kohanová D. The impact of bridging education programs on internationally educated nurses becoming registered nurses in high-income countries: a mixed-methods systematic review. Int Nurs Rev. 2025;72(2):e13038. https://doi.org/10.1111/inr.13038.
158. Miller P. The NHS needs to confront the serious problem of racism within the service; 2024, NHS Confederation Blog 14 Aug 2024 [cited 16.04.2025] Available from https://www.nhsconfed.org/articles/nhs-needs-confront-serious-problem-racism-within-service
159. Unison. Anti-racism in the workplace and model anti-racism policy – race for equality: challenging racism in the NHS. London: Unison; 2022.
160. Smith PA, Allan H, Henry LW, Larsden JA & Mackintosh MM, Valuing and recognising the talents of a diverse healthcare workplace: report from the REOH study: researching equal opportunities for internationally recruited nurses and other healthcare workforce. University of Surrey; 2006.
161. Tagumpay KNG. A Filipino nurse educator leads the call for inclusion in global healthcare; 2025, The Global Filipino Magazine 28 April 2025 [cited 16.04.2025] Available at https://theglobalfilipinomagazine.com/a-filipino-nurse-educator-leads-the-call-for-inclusion-in-global-healthcare/
162. Bardi JNA. Internationally educated nurses face unique hurdles and need specific support; 2024, Nursing Times 28 November Available at https://www.nursingtimes.net/workforce/internationally-educated-nurses-face-unique-hurdles-and-need-specific-support-28-11-2024/
163. Pressley C et al. Supporting internationally educated nurses to stay and thrive in the NHS; 2024, Nursing Times [online], 120; 6.
164. Mwaba NC. Stay and Thrive: Mid Yorkshire Teaching NHS Trust; 2025. [cited 16.04.2025] Available from https://www.workforcechallengehub.net/news/stay-thrive/
165. NHS England. Enabling staff movement. London: NHSE; 2024.
166. Adhikari R, Melia KM. The (mis)management of migrant nurses in the UK: a sociological study. J Nurs Manag. 2015;23:359–67. https://doi.org/10.1111/jonm.12141.
167. Fernando F. Latest update Filipino nurses 8b to Band 9 in the NHS. 2021 Tweet by @fernandof1974 https://x.com/fernandof1974/status/1359980003224600581
168. Florence Nightingale Foundation. The potential impacts of additional advanced practice regulation on internationally educated nurses and midwives in the UK: final report. London: FNF; 2024.
169. Nursing Standard. Free leader mentoring for Filipino nurses. Nurs Stand. 2021;36(5):36. https://doi.org/10.7748/ns.36.5.6.s3.

A Comprehensive Analysis of Globalization and Integration of Internationally Educated Nurses in Australia

Scott Bennett and Faustino Jerome Babate

Global Shortage

The Impact on Australia

The shortage of nurses is a complex issue that compromises the foundation of healthcare delivery of one of the highest functioning health systems in the world.[1] This commentary explores the multifaceted nature of the global nursing supply and utilisation, its specific impact on Australia, and the urgent need for comprehensive strategies to address the need.

The nursing shortage is a global phenomenon, with estimates suggesting that there will be a shortfall of 13 million nurses by 2030.[2] This shortage is driven by various factors, including ageing populations, increasing healthcare demands, and insufficient investment in nursing education and workforce planning.

In many countries, especially those that rely heavily on internationally educated nurses (IENs), the COVID-19 pandemic has exacerbated the situation, leading to increased burnout, attrition, and early retirement among nurses [1]. In Australia, the Commonwealth government's recent modelling predicts a shortfall of at least

[1] Blumenthal D, Gumas ED, Shah A, Gunja MZ, Williams II RD. 2024. A Portrait of the Failing US Health System: Comparing Performance in 10 Nations.

[2] World Health Organization. State of the world's nursing 2020: Investing in education, jobs and leadership. 2020. from: https://www.who.int/publications/i/item/9789240003279

S. Bennett (✉) · F. J. Babate
Filipino Nursing Diaspora Network, Sydney, NSW, Australia
e-mail: jerome.babate@findnetwork.org

R. El Moubadder et al. (eds.), *Globalization and Integration of Internationally Educated Nurses: A Comprehensive Analysis*,
https://doi.org/10.1007/978-3-032-01106-0_5

70,000 nurses by 2034.[3] The same study also predicts that the proportion of staff gaining their initial registration in Australia will fall from 80% to 72%. The increase in total demand heralds a substantial increase in the population of internationally qualified nurses.

Nurses are crucial in healthcare systems, providing essential care across various settings, from hospitals to community health services. The shortage of nurses has significant implications for patient care, leading to increased workloads, higher stress levels, and compromised quality of care.[4] The shortage also affects the ability of healthcare systems to respond to public health emergencies, as seen during the COVID-19 pandemic when many countries struggled to mobilise sufficient nursing resources.

With a global shortage of nurses and midwives well documented [2], Australia competes with many other health systems across the globe to recruit enough IENs to meet demand, which cannot be supplied through local training and recruitment. Moreover, the COVID-19 pandemic has complicated recruitment efforts, with travel restrictions and border closures disrupting the flow of skilled workers into Australia [3]. As this chapter will elaborate on, Australia's success in doing so will be based on its ability to maximise its attractiveness as the destination country for qualified professionals while addressing some of the severe challenges that new residents face when they arrive in Australia, including the cost of living, geographical remoteness, and the country's ability to respond and adapt to climate change. This is a small example of how open and transparent Australian healthcare providers are in seeking internationally trained nurses to obtain the best-qualified staff to meet the current demand.

Nurses and midwives comprise more than half of Australia's health workforce—and almost 90% are women.[5] Australia has a strong tradition of recruiting health professionals internationally, including nurses and midwives [4]. The country has been grappling with a shortage of nurses for several years, and the situation is expected to worsen as the demand for healthcare services continues to rise.

Several factors contribute to the nursing supply and demand mismatch in Australia. The ageing population is one of the most significant drivers, leading to increased demand for healthcare services, particularly in aged care and chronic disease management. Additionally, the nursing workforce itself is ageing, with a large proportion of nurses approaching retirement age. This demographic shift is creating a gap that is not being filled quickly enough by new graduates.

The shortage of nurses, particularly those with specialised skills, severely affects patient care. Issues such as delayed diagnoses and postponed surgeries directly result from these shortages, especially in areas like paediatric emergency

[3] Department of Health and Aged Care, Commonwealth of Australia, 2024. Nursing Supply and Demand Study 2023–2035. Canberra.

[4] International Council of Nurses. (2021). International Nurses Day 2021: Nurses: A Voice to Lead—A Vision for Future Healthcare.

[5] Together, nurses and midwives make up more than half of Australia's health workforce - and almost 90 per cent are women.

departments [5]. The underutilisation of IENs' skills due to credential recognition issues further exacerbates these problems, leading to inefficiencies and reduced quality of care.

Economically, the nursing shortage poses significant challenges. High attrition rates among nurses, particularly IENs, due to dissatisfaction and deskilling lead to increased recruitment, training, and retention costs [6]. Additionally, reliance on agency staffing to fill gaps inflates the operational costs of healthcare providers, impacting their financial stability and ability to invest in long-term improvements [7].

Australia will also need to be acutely aware of the unintended consequences of recruiting IENs, including an under-investment in the development and training domestically and creating nursing skill shortages in developing health economies. Recruiting nurses from countries with workforce shortages can exacerbate global inequalities in healthcare access. Australia has committed to ethical recruitment practices to address this issue, including adherence to the World Health Organization's Global Code of Practice on the International Recruitment of Health Personnel. This code emphasises the need to balance the benefits of international recruitment with the responsibility to support the development of local health systems in source countries.[6]

Immigration

Recruitment

Australia's health system recruits skilled migrants to fill labour shortages, particularly in the healthcare, engineering, and information technology sectors. Skilled migration is a response to workforce demands and a strategic tool for fostering innovation and economic growth. The skilled migration programme, which includes the general skilled migration (GSM) stream and employer-sponsored visas, is central to this effort.

To better understand the recruitment process, IENs need to know how the health system is organised and how the nursing profession is structured.

The Structure of the Health System

The Australian health system is a blended public and private system with universal access to all Australians. Responsibilities for funding and provision of care are split between the Commonwealth government and state/territory governments. Each

[6] Health Workforce (HWF. WHO Global Code of Practice on the International Recruitment of Health Personnel [Internet]. Who.int. World Health Organization; (2010). https://www.who.int/publications/i/item/who-global-code-of-practice-on-the-international-recruitment-of-health-personnel

state/territory organises their acute health systems. For example, Victoria, Australia's second most populous state, currently has 73 health services, a collection of hospitals and community services. Each health service operates its own recruitment, making navigating the process complex. By comparison, New South Wales, Australia's largest state, collects its hospitals and acute community services into 15 local health districts and operates local and single-point recruitment.

The Commonwealth government is responsible for primary care, with most general practitioners operating as "small businesses", a blend of for-purpose, public, and private providers supporting nursing and midwifery services in primary care.

Aged care is also the responsibility of the Commonwealth, which has a blend of private, for-purpose, denominational, and public providers.

As part of the multidisciplinary team, nurses work across many settings, including:

- Aboriginal Community Controlled Health Services.
- Public and private hospitals.
- Aged care (both residential and home).
- Primary care practices, including general practice.
- Community health services.
- Schools.
- Correctional facilities.
- Rural and remote communities.

More information on the organisation, size, and rich data sources in all jurisdictions in Australia is available from the Australian Institute of Health and Welfare.[7]

The Structure of the Profession

In Australia, nurses are regulated health professionals who complete approved training pathways to register with the Nursing and Midwifery Board of Australia (NMBA). The NMBA collaborates with the Australian Health Practitioner Regulation Agency to regulate nursing. Registration with the NMBA is required to use the titles:

- Assistant in nursing.
- Enrolled[8] nurse.
- Registered nurse.
- Nurse practitioner.

Assistants in nursing are a relatively new part of the nursing professional family in Australia. They are often nursing students and work in addition to the other

[7] https://www.aihw.gov.au/reports/australias-health/health-system-overview

[8] Summarised from https://www.health.gov.au/topics/nurses-and-midwives/about

prescribed ratios or staffing levels. Nursing in Australia relies much less heavily on the nurse assistant or auxiliary nurse role than systems like the United Kingdom.

Enrolled nurses (ENs) complete a vocational nursing diploma through a vocational education provider. ENs work under the supervision of a registered nurse and cannot act alone. ENs can become an RN through additional training. With a nursing team led by an RN, EN's duties generally include:

- Recording patients' vital signs.
- Administering treatments and medicines from care plans.
- Assisting with health education activities.
- Collaborating in multidisciplinary teams.
- Supporting patients with daily activities.

Registered nurses (RNs) complete either a 3-year undergrad or 2-year postgrad masters with a minimum of 750 clinical placement hours through a university. RNs graduating in Australia often undertake a graduate year with a structured, supported transition to practice. These programmes frequently involve orations between clinical environments to support the transition to clinical practice; however, they are not mandatory.

- Assess, plan, and implement nursing care to meet a patient or user's needs.
- Administering medicines.
- Supervising ENs and junior RNs.
- Providing specialised nursing care.
- Undertaking regular professional development.
- Performing leadership and management roles.
- Working in advanced or highly specialised practice.

Nurse practitioners (NPs) are RNs whom the NMBA have endorsed as an NP by the NMBA. NPs practice independently in advanced and extended clinical roles and can prescribe medicines within the scope of their practice.

To be eligible for an NP endorsement, a nurse must:

- Be a registered nurse with no restrictions on practice.
- Have 5000 hours of experience at the advanced clinical nursing practice level in the past 6 years.
- Have completed an approved programme of study at a master's degree level.
- Comply with the NMBA's nurse practitioner standards for practice.

State and territory governments employ most NPs in acute care settings. Private settings also employ NPs as employees or in their own practice.

Policies

Australia's immigration policies are designed to balance the need for skilled labour with protecting national interests. The country's highly regulated immigration system includes points-based assessments, employer sponsorship, and state or territory nominations. These mechanisms ensure that immigrants possess the skills, qualifications, and English language proficiency required to contribute to the economy.

The points-based system, introduced in the late twentieth century, is one of the key features of Australia's immigration policy. It assesses potential migrants based on age, education, work experience, and language skills. This system is designed to attract young, highly educated individuals who can integrate quickly into the Australian workforce. However, critics argue that the points system can be overly restrictive and may overlook the contributions of older or less formally educated migrants who still possess valuable skills and experience.[9]

Employer-sponsored visas, such as the Temporary Skill Shortage (TSS) visa and the Employer Nomination Scheme (ENS) visa, provide a more direct pathway for skilled workers to enter Australia. These visas allow employers to sponsor foreign workers for positions that cannot be filled locally. While these visas have effectively addressed immediate labour shortages, they also raise concerns about worker exploitation and the potential for wage suppression. To mitigate these risks, the Australian government has implemented stricter labour market testing requirements and introduced measures to protect the rights of migrant workers.

Migration trends have shifted significantly in recent years, with a growing emphasis on regional migration. The Regional Migration Scheme encourages skilled migrants to settle in areas outside the major cities, where labour shortages are often more acute. This policy aims to address the uneven distribution of the population and stimulate economic development in regional Australia. However, attracting and retaining migrants in regional areas remains a challenge, as many prefer to live in metropolitan regions where job opportunities and services are more readily accessible.

Future Directions

The Australian government has implemented several policy responses to address the challenges and opportunities associated with immigration. These policies aim to balance the need for skilled labour with the protection of national interests and the rights of migrants. Key policy areas include:

1. *Streamlining Visa Processes*: The government has introduced measures to simplify visa processing for skilled migrants, particularly in critical sectors such as

[9] Birrell B. Australia's skilled migration program: scarce skills not required. Monash University, VIC: The Australian Population Research Institute. At https://www.macrobusiness.comau/wpcontent/uploads/2018/03/Final-March-8-Australias-skilled-migration-program-1.pdf. 2018 Mar.

healthcare. This includes priority processing for occupations on the Skilled Occupation List (SOL) and reducing the complexity of visa applications.
2. *Supporting Regional Migration*: To address the uneven distribution of migrants, the government has implemented initiatives to encourage settlement in regional areas. These include the Regional Sponsored Migration Scheme (RSMS) and the Designated Area Migration Agreements (DAMAs), which provide additional incentives for migrants to live and work in regional Australia.
3. *Enhancing Worker Protections*: In response to concerns about the exploitation of temporary migrants, the government has introduced measures to protect the rights of migrant workers. This includes strengthening labour market testing requirements, increasing penalties for employers who violate labour laws, and providing support services for migrant workers.
4. *Facilitating Pathways to Permanent Residency*: Recognizing the contributions of temporary migrants, the government has introduced clearer pathways to permanent residency. This includes expanding the eligibility criteria for permanent visas and reducing the barriers to transitioning from temporary to permanent status.
5. *Promoting Ethical Recruitment*: Australia is committed to ethical recruitment practices, particularly in the healthcare sector. This includes adherence to international codes of practice and collaboration with source countries to ensure that recruitment does not undermine local healthcare systems.

Looking to the future, Australia's immigration policies must continue to evolve in response to changing global dynamics and domestic needs. This includes addressing the challenges of an ageing population and ensuring sustainability.

Migration

Migration trends in Australia have evolved, reflecting changes in global migration patterns, domestic labour market needs, and government policies. Historically, Australia's migration programme was dominated by European migrants, but this has shifted towards Asia and other regions in recent decades. Today, migrants from countries such as India, China, and the Philippines represent a significant proportion of Australia's immigrant population.[10]

One of the most significant shifts in migration trends has been the increasing focus on temporary migration. Temporary visa holders, including international students, working holidaymakers, and temporary skilled workers, now comprise a substantial portion of the migrant population. These migrants contribute to the economy, particularly in agriculture, hospitality, and healthcare sectors. Still, they also face challenges related to job security, access to services, and pathways to permanent

[10] Australian Bureau of Statistics. Cultural diversity: Census, 2021 [Internet]. www.abs.gov.au. Australian Bureau of Statistics; 2022. Available from: https://www.abs.gov.au/statistics/people/people-and-communities/cultural-diversity-census/latest-release

residency [8]. To address these concerns, the Australian government has introduced measures to strengthen the rights of temporary migrants and provide clearer pathways to permanent residency.

The rise of temporary migration has also sparked debate about the long-term impacts on Australian society. Critics argue that the reliance on temporary migrants can create a two-tiered labour market, where temporary workers are vulnerable to exploitation and have limited rights compared to permanent residents and citizens.[11]

Another challenge facing Australia's migration programme is the integration of migrants into the workforce and broader society. While Australia has a relatively successful track record of integrating migrants, there are ongoing concerns about discrimination, underemployment, and social exclusion. Migrants, particularly those from non-English-speaking backgrounds, often face barriers to employment, such as the non-recognition of overseas qualifications, language barriers, and discrimination [9].

Entry into Australia

For Australian and New Zealand citizens living aboard, entry into Australia is straightforward, with no visas required to enter or reside in the country. Suppose you qualify for a visa category such as a partner or spouse visa. In that case, you must consider obtaining a visa aligned to your skills and qualifications through the general skilled migration programme[12] to enter the country as a skilled migrant. This programme has been designed to attract migrants who can contribute significantly to Australia and fill positions without local workers. This is particularly relevant in regional areas of the country, which have traditionally struggled to recruit and retain locally trained and qualified nurses and midwives. The programme is deliberately dynamic to flex to the changing economic and employment demands, so it is essential for anyone considering applying as an IEN in Australia to stay abreast of any changes to the programme.

One of Australia's most significant aspects of its recruitment strategy is its focus on targeted occupations. The Department of Home Affairs maintains a Skilled Occupation List (SOL), identifying professions in high demand nationwide. This list guides the recruitment of skilled migrants, ensuring that immigration aligns with the labour market. For example, the persistent nursing shortage has led to the inclusion of registered nurses on the SOL, making them eligible for priority processing and offering incentives to attract international talent.

The Australian Nursing and Midwifery Accreditation Council (ANMAC) is the independent organisation gazetted (appointed) by the Federal Minister for

[11] Parliament of Australia, https://www.aph.gov.au/Parliamentary_Business/Committees/Joint/Migration/MigrationPathway/Report/Chapter_7_-_Skilled_Migration

[12] Australian Government Department of Home Affairs. Skilled migration program [Internet]. Homeaffairs.gov.au. 2019. Available from: https://immi.homeaffairs.gov.au/what-we-do/skilled-migration-program

Immigration to perform skills assessment for migration purposes under this programme[13] for professions falling under the banner of nursing or midwifery. The ANMAC considers work experience in assessing an applicant's qualifications, which is then used to determine suitability for skilled migration.

The type of visas available for each occupation on the list will have their specific requirements. By way of example, as of the date of publication, qualified nurses are eligible to apply for the following[14]:

- *186—Employer Nomination Scheme visa (subclass 186)*
- *189—Skilled Independent (subclass 189)—points-tested*
- *190—Skilled Nominated (subclass 190)*
- *407—Training visa (subclass 407)*
- *485—Temporary Graduate (subclass 485)—graduate work*
- *489—Skilled Regional (Provisional) visa (subclass 489)—family-sponsored*
- *489—Skilled Regional (Provisional) visa (subclass 489)—state or territory nominated*
- *482—Temporary Skill Shortage (subclass 482)—medium-term stream*
- *187—Regional Sponsor Migration Scheme (subclass 187)*
- *494—Skilled Employer Sponsored Regional (provisional) (subclass 494)—employer-sponsored stream*
- *491—Skilled Work Regional (provisional) visa (subclass 491)—state or territory nominated*
- *491—Skilled Work Regional (provisional) visa (subclass 491)—family-sponsored.*

Mobilisation

Australia's economy heavily relies on recruiting skilled migrants to fill labour shortages, particularly in the healthcare, engineering, and information technology sectors. Skilled migration is a response to workforce demands and a strategic tool for fostering innovation and economic growth. The skilled migration programme, which includes the general skilled migration (GSM) stream and employer-sponsored visas, is central to this effort.

Australia's immigration programme is biased towards filling roles that domestically qualified workers cannot fill. There is a significant disparity between urban and rural areas, with rural and remote regions facing more severe shortages. Nurses

[13] Nursingmidwiferyboard.gov.au. 2024 [cited 2024 Dec 8]. Available from: https://www.nursingmidwiferyboard.gov.au/Accreditation/IQNM/Before-you-apply/Immigration-and-employment.aspx#)

[14] Australian Government. Skilled occupation list [Internet]. Homeaffairs.gov.au. 2019. Available from: https://immi.homeaffairs.gov.au/visas/working-in-australia/skill-occupation-list

in these areas often work in challenging conditions with limited resources, leading to higher turnover rates and difficulty attracting new staff.[15]

While nursing registration in Australia is nationally regulated under the Australian Health Practitioner Regulation Agency (AHPRA) and the Nursing and Midwifery Board of Australia (NMBA), allowing nurses to practice across all states and territories without the need for additional licensure, practical barriers to state-to-state mobility can still exist. Differences in enterprise bargaining agreements, award conditions, rostering practices, and entitlements such as salary packaging, leave arrangements, and professional development access can influence a nurse's decision to relocate. In some cases, nurses may face variations in onboarding requirements, local policies, or hospital-specific credentialing, especially in highly specialized practice areas. Despite these differences, the unified national registration system remains a significant enabler of workforce flexibility and supports the rapid deployment of nursing staff to areas of critical need, including during public health emergencies or disaster response.

Healthcare Context

First Nations Australians

When moving to Australia, you must be aware of the history and contemporary opportunities and challenges of Aboriginal and Torres Strait Islander people. First Nations Australians are considered the custodians of the longest continuing culture in the world. Since colonisation, there has been a long history of disposition and racism that pervades even the healthcare sector.[16]

According to the Australian Bureau of Statistics, as of 30 June 2021, 983,700 Aboriginal and Torres Strait Islander people live across the country. Australia's First Nations people are made up of many different and distinct groups, each with their own culture, customs, language, and laws, and are considered the world's oldest surviving culture.

First Nations people's health outcomes are significantly lower than those of other Australians. As such, a number of programmes are established to seek improvement in these outcomes, as well as the delivery of health in a manner that aligns with and respects cultural traditions.

Indigenous Australians experience lower life expectancy, higher rates of chronic disease, and reduced access to healthcare services. Efforts to close the gap in health outcomes between Indigenous and non-Indigenous Australians have been a national

[15] AIHW. (2022). Nursing workforce. Australian Institute of Health and Welfare. https://www.aihw.gov.au/reports/workforce/nursing-workforce/contents/nursing-workforce

[16] Australian Institute of Health and Welfare. Cultural safety in health care for Indigenous Australians: monitoring framework [Internet]. Canberra: Australian Institute of Health and Welfare, 2023 [cited 2024 Dec. 9]. Available from: https://www.aihw.gov.au/reports/indigenous-australians/cultural-safety-health-care-framework

priority for many years, but progress has been slow.[17] Addressing these disparities requires a multifaceted approach that includes improving access to culturally appropriate healthcare, addressing the social determinants of health, and involving Indigenous communities in the design and delivery of health services [10].

You are likely to find a dedicated First Nations unit or leader within the organisation you work with and a requirement to complete dedicated training to support culturally safe and appropriate care.

The Role of Technology and Innovation in Australian Healthcare

Technology and innovation are increasingly important in shaping the future of healthcare in Australia. Integrating digital health technologies, such as electronic health records (EHRs), telemedicine, and mobile health applications, can potentially improve the efficiency and accessibility of healthcare services. These technologies are particularly valuable in addressing the challenges of delivering care in rural and remote areas, where geographic barriers can limit access to healthcare.

Telemedicine, in particular, has seen significant growth in Australia, driven by the need to provide care during the COVID-19 pandemic. Telehealth consultations have become a critical tool for ensuring continuity of care, allowing patients to access medical advice and treatment without needing in-person visits. This shift has been supported by government policies that have expanded the scope of telehealth services under Medicare, making them more widely available to the population.

However, the adoption of digital health technologies also presents challenges. These include data privacy and security issues, the digital divide (particularly among older adults and low-income populations), and the need for healthcare professionals to develop new skills to use these tools effectively. Ensuring that the benefits of digital health are equitably distributed will require targeted policies and investment in digital literacy and infrastructure [11].

The Future of Australian Healthcare: Strategic Directions

As Australia's healthcare system faces the challenges of an ageing population, workforce shortages, and increasing demands, strategic planning and policy development are essential to ensuring its future resilience. Several key areas require ongoing attention:

- *Workforce Planning and Development*: Addressing the nursing shortage and other healthcare workforce challenges will require a coordinated approach that includes increasing the capacity of training programmes, improving retention,

[17] Australian Institute of Health and Welfare. First Nations people and the health system [Internet]. Canberra: Australian Institute of Health and Welfare, 2024 [cited 2024 Dec. 9]. Available from: https://www.aihw.gov.au/reports/australias-health/indigenous-australians-use-of-health-services

and leveraging international recruitment ethically. Additionally, strategies to enhance the skills and competencies of the existing workforce, particularly in areas such as digital health and chronic disease management, are critical.

- *Integration of Care*: The complexity of the Australian healthcare system, with its mix of public and private providers, requires better care integration across different levels and settings. This includes improving communication and collaboration between primary care, specialist services, and hospitals and ensuring that patients receive coordinated, person-centred care.
- *Innovation and Technology*: The adoption of digital health technologies and innovative care models, such as telemedicine, must be supported by policies that address the implementation challenges, including data privacy, digital literacy, and equity of access. Investing in research and development and fostering partnerships between the healthcare sector and technology companies will be essential to driving innovation.
- *Health Equity*: Reducing health inequities, particularly for Indigenous Australians and other vulnerable populations, must remain a central focus of healthcare policy. This includes addressing the social determinants of health, improving access to culturally appropriate care, and ensuring that all Australians can benefit from the country's healthcare advancements.
- *Sustainability*: Ensuring the long-term sustainability of the healthcare system will require careful management of resources, including addressing the rising healthcare costs and the increasing burden of chronic diseases. Preventive care and public health initiatives, such as promoting healthy lifestyles and reducing the incidence of preventable diseases, are critical components of a sustainable healthcare strategy.

Integration

Integrating internationally educated nurses (IENs) into Australia's healthcare system is a critical strategy to address the nation's nursing shortage. IENs bring valuable skills, diverse experiences, and cultural perspectives that enrich the healthcare workforce. However, their integration is a complex process involving rigorous registration requirements, workplace adaptation, and community integration. This commentary explores the profile of IENs in Australia, the nurse registration process, and the challenges and opportunities associated with their integration into the workplace and community.

IEN Profile

Internationally educated nurses (IENs) represent a significant portion of the nursing workforce in Australia. These nurses come from diverse backgrounds, with the majority originating from countries such as the Philippines, India, the United Kingdom, and New Zealand. The reasons for migrating to Australia vary, but common factors include pursuing better career opportunities, higher wages, and the appeal of living in a stable and prosperous country.

IENs typically have varying experience levels, from newly qualified nurses seeking to establish careers to seasoned professionals with decades of experience in their home countries. Many IENs possess specialised critical care, mental health, and community nursing skills, which are highly valuable in Australian healthcare [12]. However, the transition to nursing in Australia can be challenging, particularly for those who must navigate a new healthcare system, cultural differences, and the demands of a highly regulated profession.

One of the distinguishing features of IENs in Australia is their linguistic and cultural diversity. Many IENs speak multiple languages and have experience working in multicultural environments, which can be an asset in providing culturally competent care to Australia's diverse population. However, this diversity can also pose challenges, particularly regarding language proficiency and the need to adapt to the cultural norms of the Australian healthcare system.

In the registration year 2023/2024, 38,816 newly registered qualified nurses and midwives were registered in Australia, making up approximately 4% of the total currently registered. A total of 16,622,[18] or 43% of this newly registered cohort, were internationally qualified. This percentage is considered high, mainly due to post-COVID healthcare demands, and will likely decrease in the short to medium term. However, integrating IENs, particularly those with specialist skills, into the healthcare system is complex and fraught with challenges, including recognising qualifications and effectively utilising their skills.

The federal government acknowledges that there will be a long-term reliance on international recruitment, with its research noting that by 2035, only 72% of nurses will obtain their initial qualification in Australia, down from the current rate of 80% (https://hwd.health.gov.au/resources/primary/nursing-supply-and-demand-study-2023-2035.pdf).

Nursing statistics as of 30 June 2023[19]:

- There were 465,993 registered nurses.
- The average age of a nurse was 43, with 33.1% aged under 35, 43% aged between 35 and 54, and 23.9% aged over 55.
- 11.9% of nurses are male.
- Nationally, there were 1760.6 nurses per 100,000 head of population (with South Australia having the highest number at 2056 and New South Wales (NSW) the lowest number at 1460).

[18] NMBA (2023a) *2023/24 annual summary, Nursing and Midwifery Board of Australia*. Available at: https://www.nursingmidwiferyboard.gov.au/News/Annual-report.aspx (Accessed: 09 December 2024).

[19] NMBA (2023b) *Health Profession Demographic Snapshot, Nursing and Midwifery Board of Australia*. Available at: https://www.nursingmidwiferyboard.gov.au/About/Health-profession-demographic-snapshot.aspx (Accessed: 09 December 2024).

Midwife statistics as of 30 June 2023[56]:

- There were 33.060 registered midwives.
- The average age of midwives was 47, with 25.3% aged under 35, 37.7% aged between 35 and 54, and 37.1% aged over 55.
- 1.3% of midwives are male.
- Nationally, there were 124.9 midwives per 100,000 head of population (with the Northern Territory having the highest at 220.9 and NSW the lowest at 104.3).

Licensure Process

There are two paths to becoming a qualified nurse or midwife in Australia (https://www.health.vic.gov.au/nursing-and-midwifery/becoming-a-nurse-or-midwife):

First is to become an **enrolled nurse.** To register, you must hold a minimum diploma from the vocational education and training (VET) sector. Typically, enrolled nurses work in emergency departments, perioperative, mental health, palliative care, mother, birthing parent, and baby care.

The second is **registered nurses and midwives.** To register, you need to be degree-qualified through the tertiary education sector. Registered nurses tend to work in intensive care, coronary care, emergency, special care nursery, oncology, and transplant care. Registered midwives work in many different practice areas, including public or private maternity services as private practice midwives, lactation services, and perinatal clinics.

Separately, all nursing students are required to be registered by AHPRA. Generally, registration is not undertaken by the individual student; instead, education providers are responsible for making sure they have provided the AHPRA, on behalf of the NMBA, with details of all students enrolled in an NMBA-approved programme of study or who are undertaking clinical training in nursing or midwifery.

IEN Nurse Registration Process: A Rigorous Pathway

Becoming a registered nurse in Australia is rigorous and involves several steps to ensure that IENs meet the high standards required for practice. The Australian Health Practitioner Regulation Agency (AHPRA) oversees the registration process. The Australian Health Practitioner Regulation Agency (AHPRA) ensures that Australia's registered health[20]practitioners are suitably trained, qualified, and safe to practise.[21] Nursing and midwifery are key parts of AHPRA's responsibilities,

[20] Nursing and Midwifery Board of Australia. Code of Conduct for Nurses [Internet]. Nursing and Midwifery Board Ahpra. 2018. Available from: https://www.nursingmidwiferyboard.gov.au/codes-guidelines-statements/professional-standards.aspx

[21] AHPRA. Australian health practitioner regulation agency [Internet]. Ahpra.gov.au. 2022. Available from: https://www.ahpra.gov.au/About-AHPRA.aspx

including but not limited to medical, dental, paramedicine, pharmacy, and psychology. The Nursing and Midwifery Board of Australia (NMBA) also plays a key role in assessing the qualifications and competencies of IENs. The NMBA also undertakes functions set by the Health Practitioner Regulation National Law, which is in force in each state and territory (the National Law). The NMBA regulates nursing practice in Australia, and one of its key roles is to protect the public. The NMBA does this by developing standards, codes, and guidelines that establish the requirements for professional and safe practice by nurses in Australia.[22]

Initial Registration: Core Requirements

The first step in the registration process is the assessment of an IEN's educational qualifications and work experience. IENs must provide evidence that their nursing education is equivalent to the standards required in Australia. This often involves reviewing their academic transcripts, course content, and clinical experience. In cases where an IEN's qualifications are not deemed equivalent, they may be required to complete additional studies or undertake a bridging programme to meet the necessary standards.

All applicants will also need to satisfy several core requirements.[23] These include:

- Criminal History: The NMBA must check an applicant's criminal history to ensure that only nurses and midwives who are suitable and safe to practise are granted registration.
- English-Language Skills: Language proficiency is another critical component of the registration process. IENs must demonstrate a high level of English language proficiency, typically by achieving a minimum score on an approved English language test such as the International English Language Testing System (IELTS) or the Occupational English Test (OET) (NMBA, 2023).
- Continuing Professional Development: Applicants need to demonstrate how they have maintained their continuing professional development; typically, this is done by demonstrating the number of hours obtained during a registration period.
- Recency of Practice: Applicants need to demonstrate how they have maintained an adequate connection with and recent practice in nursing and/or midwifery since qualifying for or obtaining registration.
- Professional Indemnity Insurance: Applicants need to demonstrate they have arrangements that secure for them for their professional practice, e.g. insurance against civil liability incurred by, or loss arising from, a claim that is made as a

[22] NMBA. Nursing and Midwifery Board of Australia - Nursing [Internet]. Nursingmidwiferyboard.gov.au. 2023. Available from: https://www.nursingmidwiferyboard.gov.au/Nursing.aspx

[23] Nursing and Midwifery Board of Australia. Nursing and Midwifery Board of Australia—Registration Standards [Internet]. Nursingmidwiferyboard.gov.au. 2016. Available from: https://www.nursingmidwiferyboard.gov.au/Registration-Standards.aspx

result of a negligent act, error, or omission in the conduct of the nurse and/or midwife.

IENs may also be required to complete a competency assessment programme (CAP) or a bridging programme. These programmes are designed to provide IENs with the knowledge and skills needed to practice safely and effectively in the Australian healthcare system. They typically include theoretical and practical components, covering the Australian healthcare context, legal and ethical considerations, and clinical practice (Health Workforce Australia, 2013).

Upon completing the CAP or bridging programme, IENs can apply for registration with AHPRA. Once registered, they are eligible to practice as a nurse in Australia. However, the journey does not end here. Newly registered IENs often require ongoing support as they transition into the workforce, and this is where the integration process becomes critical.

The Objective Structured Clinical Examination (OSCE) Process for New Registrants from Overseas

The Objective Structured Clinical Examination (OSCE) is a key component of the Australian registration pathway for certain internationally qualified nurses and midwives whose qualifications and experience are assessed as requiring further evaluation. The OSCE is administered by the Australian Nursing and Midwifery Accreditation Council (ANMAC) on behalf of the Nursing and Midwifery Board of Australia (NMBA) and is conducted at the Adelaide Health Simulation facility in South Australia—currently the sole location offering the examination.[24]

The OSCE consists of ten separate clinical stations where candidates are assessed on their practical skills, clinical reasoning, communication, and ability to deliver patient-centred care in alignment with Australian healthcare standards.[25] Each station typically lasts 10–15 minutes and may involve simulated patients, manikins, or clinical scenarios reflecting real-life practice settings such as acute care, aged care, and community health (Australian Health Practitioner Regulation Agency (AHPRA) (2024). Nursing assessment process for internationally qualified nurses and midwives. Retrieved from https://www.ahpra.gov.au). Candidates are assessed by trained examiners using standardised marking criteria based on the NMBA Registered Nurse Standards for Practice.[26]

Before attending the OSCE, candidates are advised to familiarise themselves with Australian clinical guidelines, documentation practices, infection prevention

[24] Australian Nursing and Midwifery Accreditation Council. (2024). OSCE information for candidates. Retrieved from https://anmac.org.au

[25] Nursing and Midwifery Board of Australia. (2024). OSCE examination structure and content. Retrieved from https://www.nursingmidwiferyboard.gov.au

[26] Nursing and Midwifery Board of Australia. (2016). Registered nurse standards for practice. Retrieved from https://www.nursingmidwiferyboard.gov.au

standards, and culturally appropriate communication models, all of which may differ from their country of origin [13]. The OSCE is designed to ensure that internationally educated nurses are competent not only in clinical skills but also in their ability to practise safely within Australia's legal, ethical, and cultural frameworks [14]. Upon successful completion of the OSCE, alongside meeting other registration requirements such as English proficiency and criminal history checks, candidates may proceed to full registration with the Australian Health Practitioner Regulation Agency (AHPRA) and enter the workforce.[27]

Initial Registration: Specific Endorsements

Endorsement as a nurse practitioner: As at the date of publication, when applying for endorsement as a nurse practitioner, a nurse must be able to demonstrate all of the following:

- Current general registration as a registered nurse in Australia.
- The equivalent of 3 years of full-time experience (5000 hours) at the clinical advanced nursing practice level within the past 6 years from when the NMBA receives the complete application seeking endorsement as a nurse practitioner.
- Successful completion of an NMBA-approved programme of study leads to endorsement as a nurse practitioner or a programme substantially equivalent to an NMBA-approved programme of study, which leads to endorsement as a nurse practitioner as determined by the NMBA.
- Compliance with the NMBA's Nurse Practitioner Standards for Practice.

Annual Requirements

Nurses with general or non-practising registration must renew their registration with the NMBA by 31 May each year. AHPRA manages the registration and renewal process on behalf of the NMBA. Renewed is required annually by 31 May, regardless of how long you were registered during the previous 12 months.

When renewing your registration, you must meet the following standards: criminal history, professional indemnity insurance (PII), recency of practice, and continuing professional development (CPD). You are also expected to declare any impairment likely to detrimentally affect your practice.

[27] Australian Government Department of Health and Aged Care. (2023). Pathways for internationally qualified nurses and midwives. Retrieved from https://www.health.gov.au

Workplace Integration: Navigating Challenges and Embracing Opportunities

The workplace integration of IENs in Australia is a critical factor in ensuring that they can contribute effectively to the healthcare system. However, this process is fraught with challenges, from adapting to new clinical practices and technologies to navigating workplace cultures and expectations.

One of the primary challenges for IENs is the need to adapt to the Australian healthcare system, which may differ significantly from the systems they were trained in. This includes differences in clinical guidelines, healthcare policies, and patient care practices. For example, IENs may need to familiarise themselves with Australia's patient-centred care model, emphasising collaboration between patients and healthcare providers in decision-making[42]. Additionally, using advanced healthcare technologies, such as electronic health records (EHRs) and telemedicine, may require IENs to develop new technical skills.

Workplace culture is another critical aspect of integration. IENs must navigate the dynamics of team-based care, where collaboration and communication are key to delivering high-quality patient care. Cultural differences, such as varying approaches to hierarchy, communication styles, and attitudes towards authority, can sometimes lead to misunderstandings or conflicts in the workplace. Therefore, healthcare organisations must provide cultural competency training and support to IENs and their colleagues to foster a more inclusive and supportive work environment.

Mentorship programmes have been identified as an effective strategy for supporting the workplace integration of IENs. Experienced Australian nurses can serve as mentors, providing guidance, support, and feedback to help IENs navigate the challenges of their new work environment. These programmes facilitate the professional development of IENs, help build relationships, and foster a sense of belonging within the healthcare team.

Australia's nursing workforce is highly unionised, which can influence how nursing and the workforces operates. The Australian Nurses and Midwifery Federation (ANMF) is Australia's largest union and professional nursing and midwifery organisation. Its mission is to use its collective voice to fight for members' professional, industrial, and political rights.[28] While a national union, as the employment terms and conditions are set by each state and territory government, the most vocal and recognised parts of the ANMF are the state and territory branches.

State and territory branches can be helpful when seeking out continuous professional development (CPD) opportunities, often at no cost. They also generally provide members professional indemnity insurance (PII), although there may be variations in coverage across the country. An example of the coverage provided to Queensland ANMF Branch members can be found here: https://www.qnmu.org.au/Web/Membership/Member_Benefit_Pages/MB_Professional_Indemnity_Insurance.aspx.

[28] https://anmf.org.au/

Despite the challenges, the integration of IENs also presents significant opportunities. IENs bring a wealth of experience and diverse perspectives that can enhance patient care and contribute to the overall effectiveness of the healthcare team. Their cultural competence, multilingual abilities, and experience in different healthcare systems can be valuable assets in providing care to Australia's multicultural population[42]. Additionally, IENs in the workforce can promote greater cultural awareness and sensitivity among all staff, leading to more inclusive and patient-centred care.

Community

Beyond the workplace, integrating IENs into the broader community is essential for their overall well-being and success in Australia. Community integration involves building social networks, accessing support services, and participating in cultural and community activities.

Social networks are crucial for IENs, particularly those who have left behind family and friends in their home countries. Building connections with other IENs, Australian colleagues, and local community members can provide emotional support and help IENs feel more settled in their new environment. Community organisations, cultural associations, and religious groups often play a vital role in helping IENs connect with others and navigate the challenges of settling in a new country.

Access to support services is also important for the successful integration of IENs. This includes access to housing, healthcare, education, and employment services. IENs may face challenges in finding suitable housing, particularly in areas with high demand and limited availability. Additionally, navigating the Australian healthcare system as a patient rather than a provider can be challenging, particularly for those with limited knowledge of the system or language barriers. Support services that provide information, resources, and assistance with these aspects of settlement are essential for helping IENs establish themselves in Australia.

Cultural and community activities allow IENs to engage with their local communities and share their cultural heritage. Participation in cultural festivals, community events, and volunteer activities can help IENs build relationships and contribute to the social fabric of their communities. Additionally, these activities can provide opportunities for cultural exchange, fostering greater understanding and appreciation of diversity within the community [12].

Future Directions and Challenges

Integrating IENs into the Australian healthcare system and the broader community has significant policy implications. Ensuring the successful integration of IENs requires a coordinated approach that involves healthcare organisations, government agencies, professional bodies, and community organisations.

One key policy area is supporting bridging programmes and competency assessment pathways. These programs are essential for ensuring that IENs meet Australian standards of practice and are well-prepared to enter the workforce. Funding and access to these programmes should be expanded to accommodate the growing number of IENs seeking registration in Australia.[29]

Another vital policy consideration is providing ongoing support for IENs as they transition into the workforce. Both healthcare organisations and professional bodies should encourage and support mentorship programmes, cultural competency training, and initiatives to promote workplace inclusion. These initiatives benefit IENs and contribute to the overall quality of patient care [15].

Community integration should also be a focus of policy development. Support services that address the unique needs of IENs, such as housing, healthcare, and education, should be made more accessible. Additionally, efforts to promote social inclusion and cultural exchange within communities can help create a more welcoming environment for IENs and their families [16].

Looking to the future, Australia's approach to integrating IENs must evolve in response to changing global dynamics and domestic needs. As the demand for healthcare professionals continues to grow, the successful integration of IENs will be crucial to maintaining the quality and sustainability of Australia's healthcare system.

Vignettes

Vignette 1: Filipino Nurses Moving from New Zealand to Australia

Lina (not her real name) had always dreamed of working abroad, a goal she achieved when she landed her first nursing job in Singapore right after her Philippine licensure examination. After a few years, she moved to Qatar, where the tax-free income helped her support her family back home. When New Zealand announced relaxed visa policies for healthcare workers, Lina applied and moved to Auckland with three colleagues. They embraced the slower pace of life and picturesque landscapes, but something still felt incomplete.

Her chance came through the Trans-Tasman Mutual Recognition Agreement. Moving to Australia was seamless; her New Zealand registration was recognised without requiring requalification. Lina now works in a Melbourne hospital, thriving in a multicultural team. The better pay and opportunities for career advancement cemented her decision, though she cherishes the professional journey that brought her here.

[29] https://www.nursingmidwiferyboard.gov.au/accreditation/iqnm.aspx

Vignette 2: Indian Nurses Moving from the United Arab Emirates (UAE) After (National Council Licensure Examination (NCLEX) and OSCE

Rajiv (not his real name) worked tirelessly in a busy hospital in Dubai for 8 years. Though he appreciated the cosmopolitan environment, he dreamed of providing his children a more secure future. Passing the NCLEX was his ticket to realising this dream.

With support from a recruitment agency, Rajiv prepared for and passed the OSCE in the United Kingdom. Soon after, an Australian employer offered him a role in Sydney. Adjusting to life in Australia, Rajiv is amazed at the work-life balance and quality of public education available for his kids. His wife recently began pursuing nursing, inspired by his journey.

Vignette 3: Nepali Nurses Pursuing Nursing Degrees in Australia

Sunita (not her real name) arrived in Australia on a student visa, enrolling in a diploma of aged care at a private college. Working part-time in a care home, she gained firsthand exposure to the compassionate ethos of Australian healthcare. Encouraged by her mentors, she transitioned into a bachelor of nursing programme at a regional university.

Three years later, Sunita is now a registered nurse, working in an aged care facility while saving for her master's degree. Her success story is a testament to the resilience and accessibility of Australia's nursing education pathways for international students.

Vignette 4: Filipino Nurses Recruited for Aged Care in Regional Australia

Maria (not her real name) did not expect to leave the Philippines so soon after graduating. However, she leapt when an agency offered direct placements in Australian aged care facilities. The transition was challenging—regional Australia felt worlds apart from Manila's bustling streets—but the community's warmth made her feel at home.

Maria works in a 50-bed aged care facility in rural Queensland, where she has built deep bonds with her elderly residents. She dreams of bringing her family to Australia and hopes to transition into hospital nursing 1 day. For now, she treasures the sense of purpose her role brings.

Vignette 5: Filipino and Indian Nurses Moving from the United Kingdom to Australia

Priya (not her real name), an Indian nurse specialising in paediatric care, and Ella (not his real name), a Filipino operating theatre nurse, both began their international careers in the United Kingdom. Drawn by the National Health Service (NHS)'s reputation, they found stable jobs and valuable experience. Priya loved the diversity of her London hospital, while Ella thrived in the high-paced surgical units of Birmingham. However, over the years, both felt the strain of long hours and grey winters, yearning for a change that could rejuvenate their careers and personal lives.

Ella first heard about the opportunities in Australia from a colleague who had moved to Sydney. The prospect of competitive salaries, clear career progression, and a better work-life balance was appealing. Priya, too, began researching, learning that her UK qualifications and registration would be recognised in Australia due to professional agreements between the two countries.

Their move was seamless. Priya secured a position in a Brisbane children's hospital, and Ella joined a multidisciplinary surgical team in Melbourne. They were impressed by the similarities in healthcare systems, which made the transition effortless. However, the work culture in Australia felt noticeably different—more emphasis on collaboration, flexibility, and well-being.

Beyond work, both found joy in Australia's vibrant lifestyle. Priya often visits the Gold Coast with her husband, enjoying sunny weekends at the beach. An outdoor enthusiast, Ella enjoys hiking in the Yarra Ranges and exploring Melbourne's café scene.

Their decision to move to Australia was about professional growth and a lifestyle upgrade. They have found a balance between fulfilling careers and quality time for themselves and their families. For Priya and Ella, the move has become everything they hoped for—a beautiful setting for work and life.

References

1. Buchan J, Catton H, Shaffer FA. Sustaining and retaining the nursing workforce: a call to action. International Centre on Nurse Migration; 2021.
2. Peters M. Time to solve persistent, pernicious and widespread nursing workforce shortages. Int Nurs Rev. 2023;70(2):247–53.
3. Bollyky TJ, Castro E, Aravkin AY, Bhangdia K, Dalos J, Hulland EN, Kiernan S, Lastuka A, McHugh TA, Ostroff SM, Zheng P. Assessing COVID-19 pandemic policies and behaviours and their economic and educational trade-offs across US states from Jan 1, 2020, to July 31, 2022: an observational analysis. Lancet. 2023;401(10385):1341–60.
4. Kurup C, Burston A, Miles S. Transition of internationally qualified nurses in Australia: meta-synthesis of qualitative studies. Collegian. 2023;30(2):357–66.
5. Bryant PA, Lawrence J, Boyce S, Simpson CM, Sinclair G, Chong C, Lewis P, Lee S, Hughes R, Dalton S, Lacey C. Hospital bed replacement for acute care of children at home during the COVID-19 pandemic through a hospital-in-the-home programme. Arch Dis Child. 2023;108(7):e11.

6. Bhardwaj A, Chugh D. Effectiveness of fall prevention program on nurses' knowledge and fall prevention practices. Manipal J Nurs Health Sci. 2021;7(2):3.
7. Roche MA, Duffield CM, Homer C, Buchan J, Dimitrelis S. The rate and cost of nurse turnover in Australia. Collegian. 2015;22(4):353–8.
8. Harrap B, Hawthorne L, Holland M, McDonald JT, Scott A. Australia's superior skilled migration outcomes compared with Canada's. Int Migr. 2022;60(5):91–107.
9. Chea N, Eure T, Ramirez RA, Zlotorzynska M, Blazek GT, Nadle J, Lee J, Czaja CA, Johnston H, Barter D, Kellogg M. Characteristics of healthcare personnel with SARS-CoV-2 infection: 10 emerging infections program sites in the United States, April 2020–December 2021. Infect Control Hosp Epidemiol. 2024;21:1–9.
10. Anderson K, Gall A, Butler T, Ngampromwongse K, Hector D, Turnbull S, Lucas K, Nehill C, Boltong A, Keefe D, Garvey G. Development of key principles and best practices for co-design in health with first nations Australians. Int J Environ Res Public Health. 2022;20(1):147.
11. Wakerman J, Humphreys JS. Sustainable primary health care services in rural and remote areas: innovation and evidence. Aust J Rural Health. 2011;19(3):118–24.
12. Jeon YH, Chenoweth L. Working with a culturally and linguistically diverse (CALD) group of nurses. Collegian. 2007;14(1):16–22.
13. Health Workforce Australia. Australia's health workforce series – nurses in focus. Canberra: Australian Government; 2013.
14. Jeon YH, Chenoweth L. Working with a culturally and linguistically diverse (CALD) group of nurses. Contemp Nurse. 2007;25(1–2):50–61.
15. Primeau MD, Champagne F, Lavoie-Tremblay M. Foreign-trained nurses' experiences and socioprofessional integration best practices: an integrative literature review. Health Care Manag. 2014;33(3):245–53.
16. Ohr SO, Parker V, Jeong S, Joyce T. Migration of nurses in Australia: where and why? Aust J Prim Health. 2010;16(1):17–24.

Moving Forward: Recommendations for Advancing the Integration of Internationally Educated Nurses

Rola El Moubadder, Ruth Wojtiuk, and Ruth Lee

Global Standards and Strategic Pathways for Internationally Educated Nurses (IENs) Integration: Insights from Experts Across Five Main Hosting Immigrant Countries

Healthcare systems are still recovering from the post-COVID era which exposed health disparities among underprivileged groups and amplified the frailty of healthcare systems even in developed countries. Sustaining a strong diverse nursing workforce and advancing the ever evolving nursing profession remain the main action toward improving health equities and attaining World Health Organization (WHO)'s goal of "All for Health, Health For All investment case for a safer and healthier world" [1].

The International Council of Nurses' (ICN) theme 2025 underscores the crucial connection between investing in nurses' well-being and improving global economic health which aligns with the 14th General Programme of Work (GPW14), WHO's new strategy for 2025–2028 that has been launched during WHO assembly in Geneva.

ICN reinforces the foundational role of nurses to healthcare systems, health outcomes and economic prosperities. On International Nurses Day 2025, the ICN's key message was "Our Nurses. Our Future. Caring for Nurses Strengthens Economies" urging governments and organizations to implement policies that protect nurses' rights ensuring fair compensation and providing safe working environment [2].

For decades, IENs' migration and mobility have been a consistent global trend and are on the rise as developed countries have become sought-after destinations for nurses due to economic and political instabilities in their home countries. Higher

R. El Moubadder (✉) · R. Wojtiuk · R. Lee
CARE Centre for Internationally Educated Nurses, Toronto, ON, Canada
e-mail: RMoubadder@care4nurses.org; Rwojtiuk@care4nurses.org; RLee@care4nurses.org; www.care4nurses.org

R. El Moubadder et al. (eds.), *Globalization and Integration of Internationally Educated Nurses: A Comprehensive Analysis*,
https://doi.org/10.1007/978-3-032-01106-0_6

paying jobs, career advancement opportunities and a better quality of life for themselves and their families in the countries of migration contribute to the allure. In addition, sending remittances improves the lives of their communities back home and increases their gross domestic product (GDP). Caring for IENs is not just a moral imperative by the hosting countries but a global economic strategy. By investing in IENs as an integral part of the nursing workforce, societies can achieve better health outcomes and economic growth. The ICN calls on global leaders to recognize and act upon the critical role nurses play in shaping a healthier, more prosperous future [2].

Authors from five developed countries highlighted a common theme of the "brain drain" of IENs migrating from their home countries where their care and talent are needed. However, IENs are discriminated against, working in unfavorable employment situations, and underemployed with their expertise underutilized in the hosting countries. Nevertheless, IENs are discriminated against, working in unfavorable employment situations, and underemployed with their talents underutilized in the hosting countries [3]. In addition, many more common themes were disclosed throughout the chapters. IENs face numerous challenges in the process of migration and integration into their hosting countries including recruitment inequalities compared to their domestic counterparts with equivalent credentials and qualifications as well as racial, cultural and ethnic discrimination at workplaces. In Finland and to similar extent in the other four countries, there is a noticeable difference in access to employment between domestic nurses and IENs, as well as regional differences, where IENs in rural areas might experience more challenges to integration compared to those in urban cities. Additionally, IENs in these areas often work in unfavorable conditions with limited resources and supports [4]. It has become further evident that language and communication barriers can contribute to feelings of professional and personal identity loss as IENs navigate their journey to relicensing and the relaunching their nursing career in a new healthcare system [5].

As many developed countries depend on immigrants to fill labor shortages, our Australian colleagues highlighted that Australia's economy relies heavily on recruiting skilled IENs through "The Skilled Migration Program" which includes the "General Skilled Migration" (GSM) stream. Employer-sponsored skilled migration visas are a strategic tool for fostering innovation and economic growth. The Canadian government has taken a similar approach to the pathway of immigration of healthcare professionals including nurses. However, the authors from all five countries agree that integrating IENs, particularly those with highly specialized skills, into the healthcare system in their respective countries is still complex and fraught with barriers, including recognizing qualifications and effectively utilizing their skills to their optimal potential. There are slight variations in the immigration processes, whereas some of countries such as Australia and United Kingdom streamline and integrate the immigration pathway for IENs with the licensure and integration process, while in other countries like Canada and Finland, the immigration process and licensure process are disjointed. In the United States, the immigration and licensure processes are separated.

Strategic Recommendations

Though the authors unfolded common themes to the challenges that IENs encounter through their mobilization and immigration excursion, advancing the integration and enculturation pathways of IENs remain a key collective message to governments, healthcare systems, and organizations.

To sum up, it is vital to implement policies and global guidelines that bridge borders by streamlining the immigration and credentialing processes. This will facilitate the smooth transferring of licensure across countries allowing IENs to have a fast-tracked path to practicing their profession enabling them to utilize their knowledge, skills, and talents and contribute to healthcare systems globally.

Empowering IENs

Investing in mentoring and integration programs for IENs, enabling them to thrive and flourish, can eventually result in an equal or double return on investment and highlight the added value of the diverse talents that IENs bring to communities, healthcare systems, and economies. Adding to this, educating leaders in hosting healthcare system about meeting the unique needs of IENs by providing a working environment where IENs feel safe, valued, welcomed, and enculturated. IENs' well-being is no different than that of domestic nurses; however, their journey to gain a sense of belonging in a new environment while learning the nuances of their role and scope of practice can put them under immense strain affecting their ability to relaunch and advance their nursing careers.

Furthermore, organizations and healthcare systems need to consider designing customized orientations for IENs that addresses the barriers to workplace integration such as inequalities and discrimination based on cultural, racial, linguistic, and ethnic differences. Authors emphasize that failing to implement a robust two-way integration program may result in IENs' experiencing feelings of isolation and lack of self-efficacy and determination that can lead to poor patient outcomes and reduced retention as well as negatively impacting the IENs overall sense of well-being.

Strengthening Health Systems Through IENs' Diverse Expertise

With globalization and influx of immigrants, the hosting countries become more linguistically diverse. IENs represent a valuable and untapped human resource, beyond overcoming the nursing shortages challenges, to better meet the health needs of a culturally, racially, and ethnically diverse growing population in developed countries. Communicating with patients in their native language, IENs can provide more culturally competent client-centered care.

Diversity in the nursing profession improves health equities and accessibility. IENs bring a global perspective to the nursing profession in various highly specialized clinical settings, as well as in academia and research. As nurse educators and researchers, IENs contribute to the pedagogies and body of knowledge that strengthens research for diverse, ethnic, racial, and social groups.

Sustainable Workforce Integration

With the current challenge of a global nursing shortage of 5.8 million nurses, many healthcare systems are struggling to retain their nursing workforce due to the burden imposed by the shortage, a lack of resources, and limited mental health support to nurses. For IENs to be a long-term pipeline versus a short-term fix in mitigating health, human resources' crisis efforts must focus on the implementing the supports needed for their successful integration. The fact is that IENs will continue to choose to migrate and practice in the hosting country [2].

Another vital consideration by authors is implementing policies for ongoing support for IENs as they transition into the workforce. Both healthcare organizations and professional bodies should encourage and support mentorship programs, cultural competency training, and initiatives to promote workplace inclusion. These initiatives benefit IENs, contribute to building nursing capacity, and enhance the overall quality of patient care.

Community integration should also be a focus of policy development. Support services that address the unique needs of IENs, such as housing, healthcare, and education, should be made more accessible. Additionally, efforts to promote social inclusion and cultural exchange within communities can help create a more welcoming environment for IENs and their families [6].

Global Guidance on IEN Integration Aligning with WHO and ICN Frameworks

Collective action and the streamlining IENs' pathways from immigration to licensing, employment, and integration are global imperatives. Across countries, there is a disconnect between government immigration policymakers, governing licensing bodies, and employers regarding the removal of barriers.

As the various entities are involved in these entwined pathways, they still work in silos; more open, collaborative, and transparent dialogues need to happen.

Recommendations for a call for action to regulate international recruitment and fair hiring practices must include ensuring ethical lobbying efforts and responsive advocacy initiatives to safeguard the nursing workforce from "brain drain" and the loss of highly educated nursing talents from the 55 countries where IENs are needed to care for their own population. While IENs are being discriminated against, working in unfavorable employment situations, underemployed, and their talents underutilized such measures are essential if we are to retain the IEN nursing workforce, facilitate the evolution of the nursing profession, and ensure quality care. To influence healthcare reforms effectively and showcase their contribution, IENs need to be present in leadership positions with full participation in policymaking [1, 7].

References

1. World Health Organization. (2025). State of the World's Nursing. https://www.who.int/publications/i/item/9789240110236.
2. International Council of Nurses. Our nurses. Our future. Caring for nurses strengthens economies: International Nurses Day 2025 [Internet]. Geneva: ICN; 2025. [cited 2025 May 24]. Available from: https://www.icn.ch/news/icn-puts-wellbeing-nurses-centre-international-nurses-day-2025.
3. Kline R, & Warmington J, Too Hot to Handle? Why concerns about racism are not heard... or acted on; 2024, BRAP: Birmingham.
4. Kamau, S., Koskenranta, M., Isakov, T. M., Kuivila, H., Oikarainen, A., Tomietto, M., & Mikkonen, K. (2023). Culturally and linguistically diverse registered nurses' experiences of integration into nursing workforce–A qualitative descriptive study. Nurse education today, 121, 105700.
5. Ghazal, L. V., Ma, C., Djukic, M., & Squires, A. (2020). Transition-to-US practice experiences of internationally educated nurses: an integrative review. Western journal of nursing research, 42(5), 373–392.
6. Ohr SO, Parker V, Jeong S, Joyce T. (2010). Migration of nurses in Australia: where and why? Aust J Prim Health, 16(1):17–24.
7. World Health Organization. (2023). WHO Report on Global Health Worker Mobility. World Health Organization. WHO report on global health worker mobility.

MIX
Papier aus verantwortungsvollen Quellen
Paper from responsible sources
FSC® C105338

If you have any concerns about our products,
you can contact us on
ProductSafety@springernature.com

In case Publisher is established outside the EU,
the EU authorized representative is:
Springer Nature Customer Service Center GmbH
Europaplatz 3, 69115 Heidelberg, Germany

Printed by Libri Plureos GmbH
in Hamburg, Germany